HOW TO INCREASE YOUR

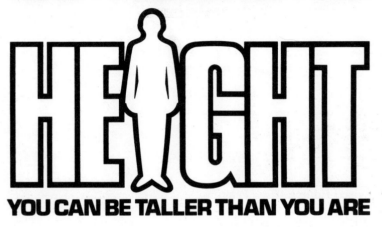

HE GHT

YOU CAN BE TALLER THAN YOU ARE

Charles W. Linart, M.D. and August Blake, with Carol B. Linart

ARCO PUBLISHING, INC.
219 PARK AVENUE SOUTH, NEW YORK, N.Y. 10003

The authors wish to acknowledge the assistance of

Mrs. Lois S. Warshauer
Human Growth Foundation
Metropolitan New York Chapter
Hicksville, New York

and

Dr. Fima Lifshitz
Chief Pediatric Endocrinologist
North Shore University Hospital
Manhasset, New York

Revised Edition, First Printing

Published by Arco Publishing, Inc.
219 Park Avenue South, New York, N.Y. 10003

Library of Congress Cataloging in Publication Data
Linart, Charles W, 1925–
　　How to increase your height.

　　1. Posture.　　2. Exercise.　　3. Stature.　　I. Blake,
August, joint author.　　II. Linart, Carol B., joint
author.　　III. Title.
RA781.5.L56　　　　　　　613.7′8　　　　　　78-8945

ISBN 0-668-04370-9 (Paper Edition)

Printed in the United States of America

Contents

Index of Figures

Preface

LIBRARIES and bookstores abound in exercise books. Repetitive exercises for physical fitness; isometric exercises to increase strength; exercises to lose weight; jogging to be fit is now enjoying popularity; yes, even exercises to improve your eyesight have in the past been published. Presented here is an exercise book, with the primary goal in mind of improving your posture and increasing your height.

In the course of my practice I have been approached by people desiring to be accepted into various institutions where there were rigid physical requirements, such as the service academies, the F.B.I., and other law enforcement agencies. These people had passed all of the other tests but were slightly lacking in one thing—height. Over the years I have assembled a series of exercises designed to accomplish this increase and in many cases the individual attained his goal.

Understand that it may not be necessary for everyone to do all of the exercises, but the more height desired, the more must be done.

Primary focus must be placed on the spine. Looking at the spine from the side, everyone sees that it has three bends; a forward curve in the neck, a backward bend in the middle and a forward curve in the lower or lumbar area. This began when man became upright in the course of the evolutionary process millions of years ago. The weight of the head—approximately

20 pounds—pressed downward on the entire spine, the weight of the arms and shoulder girdles pressed on the middle and lower spine, and the weight of the entire upper body put severe stress on the lower spine and pelvic tilt.

When a person is aging, they are known to be "shrinking" because of the increase in degree of these curves, caused largely by the length of time these pressures have been applied. If at the same time there is softening of the bones there is measurable loss of height of the individual vertebra; this is a medical problem which should be evaluated by a physician and will not be dealt with here. By decreasing the degree of the curves and straightening the spine, as a straight wire is longer than a bent one, you will be on the way to increasing your height and, incidentally, your health.

The bent wire principle also applies to the knees—bow legs and knock-knees. Though these may be improved or even corrected if caught early enough in childhood by rather simple means, once the bones have stopped growing, only rather major surgical procedures are available and are not encouraged unless the condition is extreme or causing disabling pain or joint destruction.

Many people suffer with low grade backaches, aggravated by fatigue, excessive activity, sleeping on a poor mattress or by a host of other situations. The ache is not severe, and if you have it for a long time it almost becomes a way of life. Regardless of the causes (I do not include organic, medical or orthopedic conditions), many of you will be pleasantly surprised at the disappearance of these symptoms when the exercise program is pursued diligently.

A not too uncommon situation may be seen in people who keep their knees constantly slightly bent. This can result in considerable loss of height. This involves muscles, tendons and ligaments and can be improved in the adult by some of the exercises.

I trust the book will prove enlightening and useful. Please remember that your body is the most valuable possession you have. Treat it well. In this respect periodic physical examinations are important and especially before undertaking any exercise program. It never does you any harm to see how you "stand" physically.

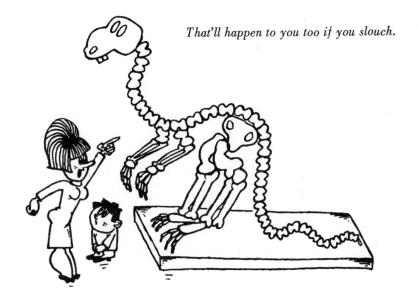

That'll happen to you too if you slouch.

Soviet Life

Introduction

SOME people may have been surprised by the following item which appeared recently in an issue of *Changing Times.**

> *My husband swears that I'm taller when I get up in the morning than when I go to bed. Can this be true?*
> There is evidence that a person can be as much as an inch shorter at dinnertime than at breakfast. The height change occurs because the spinal column relaxes and stretches during sleep and then compresses under the load of a day's activities. For some people the change is so noticeable that they have to adjust their rear-view mirrors when they drive home at night.

The above news is interesting and significant. This, however, is what really happens. It is true that an individual is taller when he awakens after a good night of sleep and rest than he is in the evening when he is ready to go to bed. During the day's activities the intervertebral discs (see figure 10) are compressed by the pressure of the vertebrae and a loss of fluid occurs. Each disc then becomes slightly thinner. The combined loss in size of all the discs add up to a shorter spine. A shorter spine means a shorter height. A loss of ½ inch in height between morning and evening would be common.

When an individual is sleeping and resting comfortably, the

---

* Courtesy of *Changing Times*, Kiplinger Magazine.

intervertebral discs reabsorb fluid and become plumper—to use a common expression—and the spine thus increases in length.

A point, then, to remember is—if you are going to take a physical examination and you want to be at your tallest, appear for the examination in the morning.

But what is more important is the fact that some people may have lost more than one inch in height permanently because of poor posture. The authors will demonstrate that it is entirely possible for an individual to increase his height. The amount that can be increased will depend upon the condition of the individual and his general muscular tone. There is a flexibility to our body, especially along the trunk or spine. This we have demonstrated in figure 1 and 2.

By exercising the proper muscles we can stretch our body and at the same time actually condition the muscles which will result in a more functional body. Many individuals are not enjoying their true potential height because of inactivity, poor posture and faulty living habits. As a result, the spine develops deeper curves than necessary. The deeper the curves, the less height one enjoys. The knees and the feet are also factors in creating conditions for loss of height.

That individuals will shrink in height has been amply demonstrated. One's mode of living, amount of exercise and general physical activity will affect a person's stature. All of us have observed a person who has had his leg or arm in a cast. When the cast is removed, the arm or leg presents a withered or shrunken look. The cast has prevented the muscles from functioning and this has caused them to shrink. Activity and exercise, however, will restore the limb to its original state.

We can apply the same analogy to our spine which although not physically broken, has, through poor posture and poor muscle development decreased in length. This poor development can actually cause a person to shrink and lose height.

For those whose height loss has been caused by poor spinal contour, the exercises outlined are designed to decrease the curvature. A straighter spine means greater height. We cannot separate our posture from the height that we enjoy. (We'll speak at this point only about posture as it concerns one's height. There are, of course, proper postures for sitting, sleeping and standing.)

If you were to pile eight boxes of assorted sizes one upon another, you would put them in such a fashion that the entire load would be utterly secure. The same is true of our body. We must carry ourselves in such a fashion so that all parts are properly balanced and that no one part puts undue stress on another. We can best illustrate this by exaggerating a condition of the body. Suppose we walk with our head tilted unduly forward. You can see how this position unbalances the body and how a lot of strain then is put on the muscles, joints and connecting tissue. If we correct this posture and bring the head back, we now have a position which produces the least amount of strain for the energy expended. If we maintain our faulty posture, in due time problems will appear. We may start complaining of backaches and other ailments.

We must remember that when we throw one part of the body out of kilter, other parts of the body make adjustments; when we position one part incorrectly, other parts also take an incorrect position. We cannot separate one part from another. When our posture is correct, breathing is easier, the amount of energy we use is less, and the stress on various parts of the body is less. Frequently when people have headaches, arthritis, backaches, or even heart trouble, the cause may go back to bad posture.

To correct our posture, exercise can play a vital role. All parts of the body are supported by muscles and unless they are in good condition, we cannot maintain a good posture. You can check your own posture by looking in a mirror or by setting up a plumb line and having someone else observe you. There are numerous books on posture which would be wise to consult. The exercise program which is designed to straighten your spine to its maximum efficient length will also improve your posture.

All sorts of bodily ills are due to poor posture. To improve

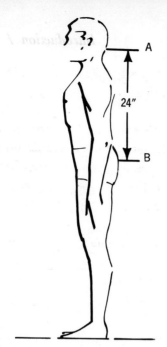

A. Spinal column measured between points A and B with a tape.
Measure equals 24 inches.

Figure 1

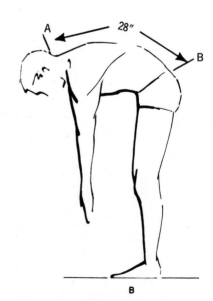

B. Spinal column measured between points A and B with a tape.
Measure equals 28 inches.

Figure 2

your posture you must strengthen your abdominal muscles in conjunction with your back muscles, since all muscles work together.

The exercises in this book were originated to remove any unnecessary curvature in the spine—to create a supple vibrant spine and to help an individual gain his full potential height.

If there is any "slack" that can be taken up, these exercises are designed to help do the job. Figures 1 and 2 illustrate the flexibility of the spine.

In order to show how much flexibility there is in the spine, do the following:

1. Stand erect as in figure 1 and have someone measure your spine from the base of the skull (point A) to the coccyx (point B).
2. Bend forward as far as you can (figure 2) without undue strain and without bending the knees.
3. Measure the spine in the new position. The difference in length, usually around four inches, between the two positions demonstrates the stretch in your spine and its flexibility.

The exercises in general have been numbered in sequence of difficulty. If your problem lies in all areas begin with #1 in each group and master it before moving on. If you feel that one area requires more attention than others concentrate on those exercises, but do some of the others in order to keep the body in balance. All exercises described must be performed daily for a minimum of six weeks and up to six months or longer. They should not be performed less than one hour after a meal or less than one hour before retiring. Do not continue any exercises beyond the feeling of discomfort, undue fatigue, or pain.

1. Posture

WHAT we possess in terms of mental and physical qualities (including height) is brought about through a combination of heredity and environment. Our basic characteristics are inherited but there is enough leeway in what we have inherited so that environmental factors can produce significant changes. Thus we cannot really separate heredity and environment and deem one more important than the other.

When we think of posture, we find that roots go back deep into our history as human beings. We find that many forces impinge on our human structure. The young infant, even before he is born, is having his posture formed in his mother's womb. The state of the mother's health, her nutrition, is affecting the baby. While in the majority of cases there is no adverse postural position that is taken, there are situations where the position of the fetus within the mother's womb is faulty, and the start of a postural defect may have begun. We are fortunate that with modern medical facilities and the routine examinations that babies undergo in hospitals most of these defects are picked up. However, parents can never let up in keeping a watchful eye on the growing infant. The child is constantly subject to some sort of postural stress which may lead to poor posture. Even while sleeping, his posture is being formed. The mother must be on the constant alert when the baby sleeps on its stomach and puts his feet in an incorrect position—in this way he can develop pigeon toes. The now largely outmoded habit of mothers carrying babies with legs straddling her body and weight supported by arm under its buttocks has been the cause of many cases of bow legs. Diapers can be a factor in developing bowlegs or weak arches and thus create a basis for a faulty posture in the future. This is why it is wise for a mother to have the child examined periodically by a physician. The quicker we pick up a problem, the easier it is to cure it.

The child from an early age is subject to various pressures. Parents are frequently over-eager to see a child walk. Let the child develop in his own way; when he is ready to walk he will do so. To keep him on his feet for too long a time can start a damaging process which if persisted can have permanently detrimental postural effects.

Every aspect of our life is interrelated. The way we view life and the way people and events impinge on us all leave some trace on us, including our personality. There is evidence that the child who is not fondled, who is not played with or who is not payed attention to, will not develop properly. Those youngsters whom parents have abandoned and who grow up in institutions without love or affection suffer personality damage. Youngsters are quick to perceive how others view them. The child who has developed a poor posture due to some illness will illicit a certain response from people. This constant interaction will mold the individual in a certain pattern.

As the individual reaches adulthood he will already have formed a certain image of himself based on his total environmental experiences. We cannot exclude posture from being a factor in this total experience. A good posture, a commanding appearance—these are qualities that elicit high social value. A person's appearance reflects his personality. The individual who walks in a half-hearted way, without energy or purpose, with a look of dejection on his face, is not apt to inspire anyone. There is always this feedback effect involved with our posture. Others observe us and in ways subtle, or perhaps not so subtle, indicate approval or disapproval. (A striking appearance will evoke favorable impressions or comments which will then reinforce what we already think about ourselves. On the other hand, a negative reaction from someone will have a poor effect on an individual.)

Carrying our point a little further, we cannot divorce the effect emotions can have on our posture. Emotions have a definite effect on our posture. A disturbed person will reflect his condition in his face, his gait, and various body movements. Depending on the severity of the condition, we may eventually effect postural change.

A highly emotional state can disturb the chemical equilibrium or balance of our body; for example, a disturbed emotional state may cause an increase in the amount of adrenalin to pour into our body. As a result of this, the glycogen (a muscle food) is broken down, lactic acid is formed, and the muscles become fatigued and are unable to relax. When muscles get no rest, they begin to ache. If you keep aching in the back or some other part of the body, you may start to change your postural habits to accommodate to this discomfort. You may start favoring a leg because of the pain and as a result muscles may start to atrophy and eventually cause an unfavorable body posture. The ache, the pain, the poor posture becomes a way of life for many people.

If an emotional state causes an individual to overeat, he is very likely to become overweight. Obesity has a definite and harmful effect on posture. If you develop a "pot" belly, it will throw your body off balance. The weakened abdominal muscles also will throw your posture off.

Good posture is comfortable and the individual feels at ease.

The body is arranged in a number of segments—head, spine, pelvis, knees, and feet. All of these parts should be so positioned that the individual when he moves can do so with a minimum energy expenditure.

Good posture cannot be forced upon one by some admonition such as "Pull in your stomach," "Out with the chest," "Bring those shoulders back." This sort of advice does little good and, in fact, may be harmful. If you follow this advice, you will be maintaining yourself under constant strain and tension. Your muscles should keep you in a state of dynamic equilibrium so that a comfortable posture is held without wasting energy. You should not, by a constant conscious effort, have to maintain yourself in a balanced postural position.

It is well to remember that there is not just one postural position. We have a lying, sitting, and standing posture and to these we give the name static since there is no movement. We also have a posture of movement—walking, running—and this we call dynamic posture. Each posture position exerts an effect on us. The importance of these positions will be discussed at some length in another section of this book.

A brace or some support should not be worn to maintain an erect and correct posture. The muscles should do the job. Wearing a brace or other type of support, unless medically called for, is actually weakening the body. If you let some gadget take over, your muscles will atrophy and your postural condition worsen.

Although we may criticize some modern styles, there are some that have been a boon to good posture. The miniskirt, for example, has made women even more aware of good posture. All of the postural defects that man is heir to come under much closer scrutiny when they are bared to full view. The theater of the nude, for example, may not become fully accepted because there is something singularly unattractive in the star who may prance out with a case of flat feet or some other visually observable defect. Of course if the trend to nudity continues, everyone will have to look at his posture with additional scrutiny.

From early life to maturity there are activities that are appropriate for each age level. If we exceed the capacity of our body to handle any exercise, movement, or activity, then we do so with a definite risk that injury may result. We will not go into a detailed account of all the activities at the various age levels that may cause injury. We certainly know by simply reading the newspapers that even those athletes who are in excellent physical condition are still open to severe injury. If this is true of those who try to maintain an excellent physical condition, we can imagine what could happen to those of us who are barely in fair condition. In this respect teachers in school, especially those who are engaged in physical education, have a special responsibility. They must choose and direct that type of activity and exercise which is appropriate to the child and his physical ability.

We must remember that an individual's posture has a great deal to do with the way a person's internal organs function. Poor posture can impede the function of the heart, lungs, and circulation. A curvature of the upper spine, round shoulders and a forward head will decrease the ability of the heart and lungs to function properly. A deep curve in the lower spine will make a youngster more prone or susceptible to a spinal injury.

It is fortunate that today many physical defects that passed unnoticed years ago, are now being detected. Regular physical examinations can detect problems that may be correctable if treated early.

It is important that individuals engage in a balanced exercise program. Overactivity of one group of muscles or a part of the body may prove harmful. Some tennis players, for example, have developed one arm to the point where it is noticeably larger than the other. Also, there is an ailment called "tennis elbow" which is an inflammation of the tendons on the outer side of the elbow, usually resulting from irritation and overuse.

If the upper trunk is overdeveloped, it may increase the dorsal curve and the forward head condition. The harmful effects of this may not be noticed until many years have passed.

Weight lifting, properly supervised, is an excellent way of developing muscles. There are, however, some movements which can definitely be harmful. Such a movement is the deep knee bend. The knee was not designed to take the type of punishment it is so often subjected to. It is bad enough to do deep knee bends without any additional weight, but when we add pound-age we compound the crime. The stress that is put on the muscles, ligaments, and cartilage in this maneuver is fantastic: the mechanical force required to bring the body from a deep knee bend to an upright position is tremendous. It is true that this exercise will develop powerful leg muscles, but you may ruin your knees in the process. A knee injury, especially if severe, may leave permanent damage. Damage to the knee and surrounding tissue may affect the way you walk and eventually your entire posture. We must always keep in mind how the body makes compensations because of a disturbance or poor alignment. The compensation that is made may very likely be producing an additional stress and strain.

The pregnant woman and the young mother should be aware of how posture effects them. Simply being pregnant eventually starts a process of tilting a woman and throwing her off balance: some women add to this unbalancing by wearing high heels. In this position she is subject to falls a lot easier. After childbirth, the posture again demands attention: the little "pot" that has developed may remain unless an exercise program to correct it is pursued. If this abdominal area is not taken care of, poor posture will continue and extend to other parts of the body.

2. The Plumb Line

You may have heard of the "plumb line" in relation to the work of carpenters or builders who use it to find an exact or absolute vertical direction. The plumb is usually a weight of lead at the end of a string. A plumb line is also used to check on our posture to see if it is properly aligned. With this measuring device we can see how far our posture has drifted from the norm. Basically, there are four positions of the body that we can use a plumb line on—front, back, the right side, and left side of the body. We've mentioned how the body is actually a number of segments. The most important area is the pelvis. The angle of the pelvic tilt, whether backward or forward is of crucial importance since the alignment of the body above and below depends upon it. We must remember that the pelvic girdle supports the spine and all that is attached to it and below it; the pelvis acts as an attachment for the lower limbs. In this flexible arrangement the pelvic position is vital.

In order to drop the plumb line, there must be some fixed position. Our body has one firm base—the foot. When the line drops it must fall just slightly in front of the ankle bone; no other area of the body can be used as a base since its position may change.

In an ideal postural situation the plumb line would pass through the following points:

1. Ear Lobe
2. Shoulder Joint
3. Hip Joint
4. Knee Joint
5. Just slightly in front of the Ankle Bone.

There are probably very few people who have an ideal posture; but it might be worthwhile to check your own posture

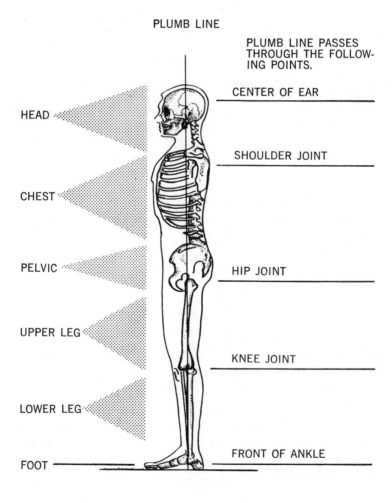

PLUMB LINE

PLUMB LINE PASSES THROUGH THE FOLLOWING POINTS.

CENTER OF EAR

HEAD

SHOULDER JOINT

CHEST

PELVIC

HIP JOINT

UPPER LEG

KNEE JOINT

LOWER LEG

FRONT OF ANKLE

FOOT

Figure 3

against this ideal. In this day of instant photography with the Polaroid camera, you can check on your posture very easily. Drop a plumb line from the ceiling or some projection above your head. Now step alongside so that the weight is just ahead of the ankle bone and see how your alignment is compared to the ideal.

In figure 3 we have an illustration of the plumb line drawn against an ideal alignment and in figure 4 we see a faulty alignment.

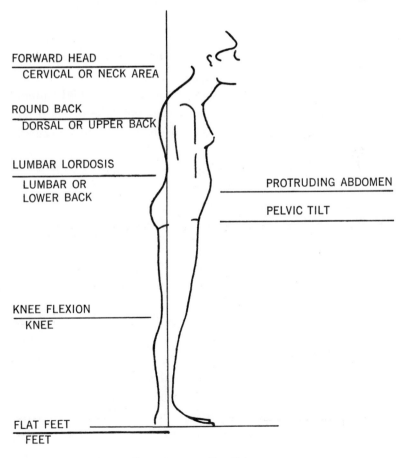

FORWARD HEAD
CERVICAL OR NECK AREA

ROUND BACK
DORSAL OR UPPER BACK

LUMBAR LORDOSIS
LUMBAR OR
LOWER BACK

PROTRUDING ABDOMEN

PELVIC TILT

KNEE FLEXION
KNEE

FLAT FEET
FEET

Lordosis   Compensatory Conditions

Figure 4

When we look at the subject in figure 4 we can at least take this positive note: there is plenty of room for improvement in posture and for an increase in height. Unfortunately, an individual with the type of postural defects illustrated is not only suffering from poor posture, but she is very likely in poor physical condition as well.

The faulty body alignment causes muscle strain, fatigue, and an overall poor physical appearance.

Pelvic Tilt

The pelvis, which really means bowl, is a key area in the body which is instrumental in maintaining balance and alignment.

The pelvic girdle is attached, at the top, to the spinal column and, at the bottom, to the thigh bone or femur. The pelvis is not stationary or static. It has a forward and backward movement and also some sideways movement. This being so, its tilt or movement, either forward or backward, will have an effect on the limbs below it and on the structure above it.

Now it is plain to see that if the pelvic girdle moves or rotates forward, then the spinal column which is attached to it must also move forward. Can it be otherwise? Now, if the lower spine moves forward, we get additional curvature. (See figures 3, 20, 21.) Note again the difference in length between the same two points when it is curved and when the curve is reduced. In our exercise program, we have carefully planned an activity that will bring into play the psoas muscle which pulls the pelvic girdle backward and thus reduces the lordosis. Some people think that all they need to do is strengthen their back to correct any difficulty. Nothing could be further from the truth. For example, ordinary ditch digging exercises the sacrospinalis muscle which pulls the lower spine forward and increases the lordosis or curvature.

Please remember that the pelvic tilt in itself does not have any effect on height; it is how the tilt affects the body above and below that may reduce height.

The exercises in figure 5 and figure 6 are designed to keep the pelvic tilt in correct alignment.

PELVIC TILT EXERCISE 1

1. Stretch body with back to floor.
2. Keep arms at side.
3. Bring both heels close to buttocks.
4. Tighten abdominal muscles as you press small of back to the floor.
5. Hold to a slow count of three.
6. Relax.
7. Work up to ten daily.

Pelvic Tilt Exercise 1

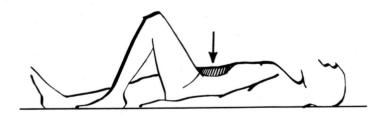

Figure 5

PELVIC TILT EXERCISE 2

This exercise should not be done until Pelvic Tilt Exercise #1 can be done ten times with ease.

1. Stand with back feet against a wall, hands at side.
2. Draw in your abdomen.
3. Press small of the back against the wall.
4. Tighten buttocks.
5. Hold to a slow count of three.
6. Relax.
7. Work up to ten daily.

Pelvic Tilt Exercise 2

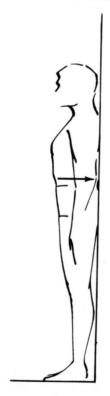

Figure 6

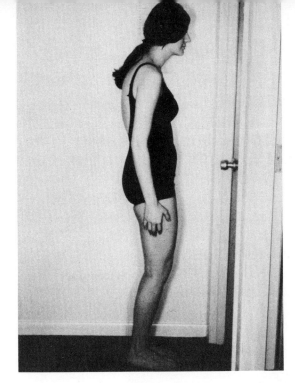

Poor Posture

Figure 7

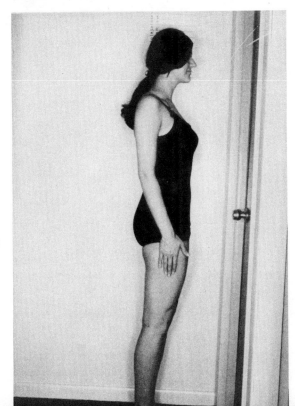

Good Posture

Figure 8

The young woman in figure 7 has lost three inches in height due to her poor or slouching posture. With her posture corrected as in figure 8, she has regained her normal height and has also assumed a more attractive posture and alignment.

Notice the forward head in the subject in the poor posture pose. If you will observe people in your daily life, notice the number that are actually walking around with their heads perched in this position. Notice also the flexed or bent knees. Again observe, when you are knee or girl watching, how many individuals are walking with their knees bent and simply pushing one leg in front of another. This situation not only causes loss of height but it's also a poor postural stance.

3. The Spine

WHEN man evolved to the upright stance he not only assumed a unique position in the animal world which enabled him to cope successfully with a hostile environment, but he also inherited a structure that contained the seeds for an assortment of difficulties and problems. Some authorities, in fact, attribute a wide variety of ailments to man's inability to successfully adjust to the upright posture.

Compared to the lower animals, man has a narrow base and supporting structure for his body. The four-legged dog, for example, has no posture problem. His four supports plant him firmly and solidly to the ground. No problem here, but this is no time to argue the merits of one position over another. Let's look at man's spine in some detail since an examination of the parts will help us understand the whole.

The spinal column (see figure 9) consists of twenty-six bones called vertebra. These twenty-six vertebra can be divided into five sections: Cervical or neck area, Thoracic or upper spine, Lumbar or lower back, Sacrum, and Coccyx. In the cervical spine there are seven vertebra. It's interesting to note, by the way, how similar we all are in the animal world. The giraffe with his long neck has seven cervical vertebrae and the whale, who looks as if he had no neck, also has seven cervical vertebrae. This cervical curve, incidentally, was one of the last to develop in the evolutionary process.

In the thoracic or upper spine there are twelve vertebrae, in the lumbar spine there are five. When an individual is born there are five distinct vertebrae in the sacrum which later unite into one. In the coccyx there are four distinct vertebrae which later unite or fuse into one.

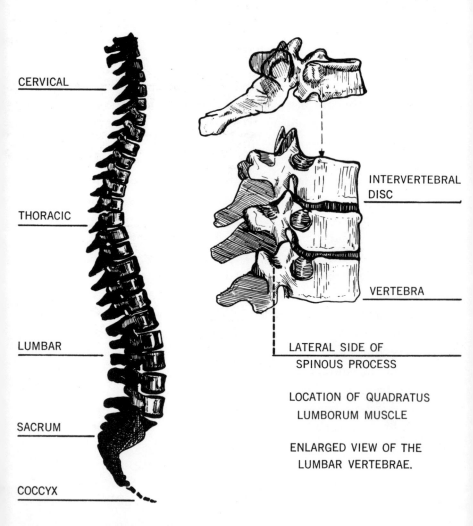

CERVICAL

THORACIC

LUMBAR

SACRUM

COCCYX

INTERVERTEBRAL DISC

VERTEBRA

LATERAL SIDE OF SPINOUS PROCESS

LOCATION OF QUADRATUS LUMBORUM MUSCLE

ENLARGED VIEW OF THE LUMBAR VERTEBRAE.

Figure 9   **Figure 10**

Please remember that it is only the general rule that there be twelve thoracic vertebrae and, as you well know, there are always exceptions to rules. You, the reader, may very well have one more or less thoracic vertebra. Our spine or body is not always as neatly packaged as illustrations and numbers would indicate. However, it is impossible to include all exceptions to the rule and the various special cases and problems to every medical or anatomical situation.

In actuality, we may think of the spine as a simple machine which performs a number of jobs with remarkable efficiency. It is a device which can be flexible and also stationary; it can move in a variety of directions; it has within itself an extremely

A curved cervical spine.

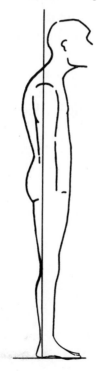

Figure 11

important cord that transmits messages. This same spinal structure also supports the body. The cervical spine supports the head; the thoracic spine supports the head plus the chest cavity and the supporting muscles and tissue. A curved cervical spine results in a forward head (see figure 11). The poor lumbar spine is left groaning at the bottom of this structure and thus must maintain all that is above plus the abdominal area which surrounds it. Is it any wonder that there are so many complaints about low back pain?

We do not mean to imply that the back is a weak structure. Far from it. However, in many ways it is a very neglected area and does not receive the care and attention that it deserves. We take the back for granted—until trouble develops.

While we are speaking of curves, please remember that the infant has only one long curve. As the child grows, it develops the three distinct curves that were mentioned in the preface of the book—a forward curve in the neck, a backward bend in the middle and a forward curve in the lumbar area.

The individual vertebra (see figure 10) are separated from each other by a disc or cushion. This arrangement allows for movement with a minimum of friction. When this cushion gives way, we have what is commonly known as a slipped disc.

4. Cervical Area

The x-ray picture in figure 12 shows the length of the cervical spine when it is curved. The length between the first cervical vertebra and the first dorsal vertebra is three inches. In figure 13 the cervical curve has been corrected and the length between the same two points is now five inches.

Courtesy of Upstate Medical Center,
Syracuse, New York

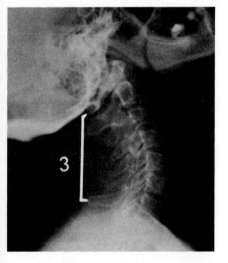 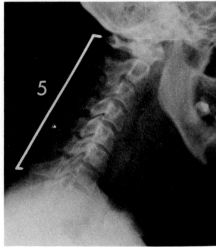

The cervical spine measured between the First cervical vertebra
and the First dorsal vertebra

Figure 12   **Figure 13**

CERVICAL EXERCISE 1

1. Lie flat on back with knees drawn up and feet flat on floor.
2. Arms are at side.
3. Draw chin inwards. Now move head upwards as you roll your neck flat against floor.
4. Hold neck to floor to the slow count of three.
5. Relax.
6. Work up to ten daily.

Cervical Exercise 1

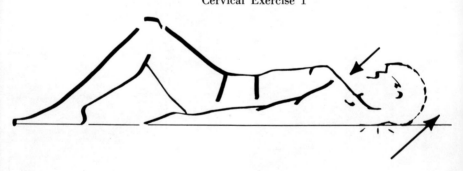

Figure 14

CERVICAL EXERCISE 2

1. Sit on a chair and clasp hands behind head. Chin down.
2. Keep elbows perpendicular to head.
3. Push head gradually against the resistance of hands.
4. Hold to a slow count of three.
5. Release gradually.
6. Relax.
7. Work up to ten daily.

Cervical Exercise 2

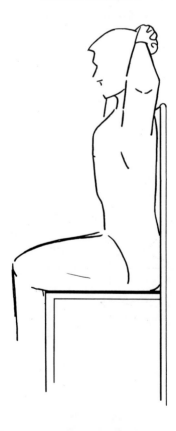

Figure 15

5. Dorsal Area

DORSAL EXERCISE 1

1. Sit on a bench or stool so that your back can be against the wall.
2. Pull in your abdomen and press lower and upper back against wall.
3. Pull in your chin and press neck and head against wall.
4. Place your hands above your head and maintain elbow contact with wall.
5. Hold to a slow count of three.
6. Now extend arms overhead in a Y position and then slowly bring hands together.
7. Relax.
8. Work up to ten daily.

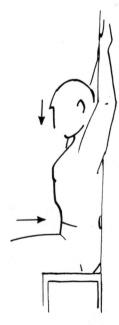

Dorsal Exercise 1

Figure 16

DORSAL EXERCISE 2

1. Lying on abdomen place forehead on the floor.
2. Raise head and upper chest as high as you can.
3. Raise legs at the same time.
4. Clasp hands together across small of back.
5. Hold to a slow count of three.
6. Lower slowly.
7. Relax.
8. Work up to ten daily.

Dorsal Exercise 2

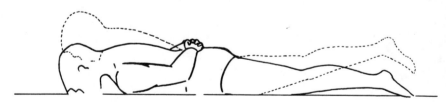

Figure 17

6. Lumbar Area

THE lumbar or lower spine exercises that follow are effective for correcting curvature in this area. The illustration in figure 18 shows a number of postural defects that may have started as

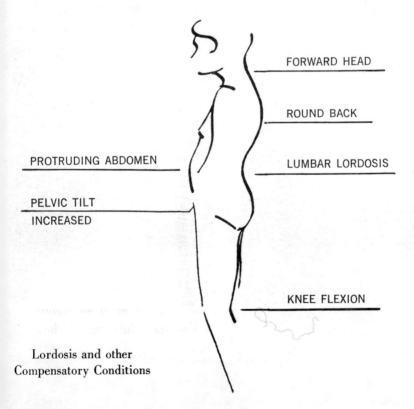

FORWARD HEAD

ROUND BACK

PROTRUDING ABDOMEN

LUMBAR LORDOSIS

PELVIC TILT
INCREASED

KNEE FLEXION

Lordosis and other
Compensatory Conditions

Figure 18

a result of a single fault. To dramatically present this problem we have actual x-ray pictures which show how curvature affects the length of the spine. When the lumbar spine is curved, the length is seven inches (see figure 19); when the curvature is reduced the length is nine inches (see figure 20). This covers the same number of vertebra—that is, the area between lumbar 1 and sacral 1. See figure 9 to get the entire perspective of the spinal column.

For those who may be unaware, the vertebrae are numbered in a certain order. For example, the topmost lumbar vertebra is referred to as number one and the bottom one is referred to as number five.

Courtesy of Upstate Medical Center,
Syracuse, New York

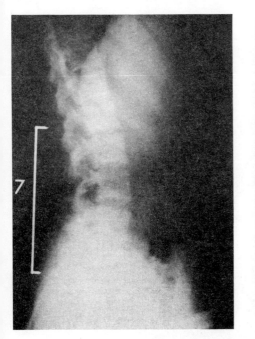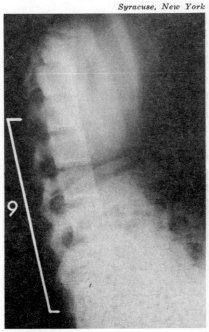

Vertebrae between lumbar 1 and sacral 1.

Figure 19   **Figure 20**

Lumbar Muscles

Note: The following exercises are extremely important in the lumbar lordosis series since they bring into play the iliopsoas and the quadratus lumborum muscles which are so vital as a stabilizing group along the spinal column. The muscular force of this group cannot consciously be felt and yet in a silent kind of way these muscles exert their important function.

The quadratus lumborum muscle is attached to the lower spine or the lumbar area. To be exact (see figures 9, 10 and 21), it is attached to the lumbar vertebrae 1, 2, 3, and 4 on the lateral side of the spinous process.

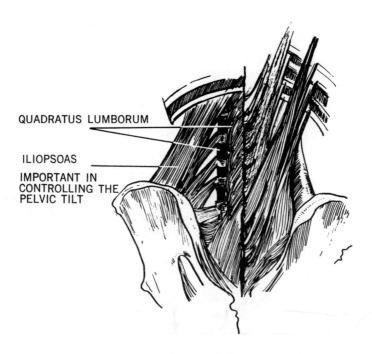

QUADRATUS LUMBORUM

ILIOPSOAS

IMPORTANT IN
CONTROLLING THE
PELVIC TILT

Figure 21

LUMBAR EXERCISE 1

1. Lie flat on your back. Feet straight and toes pointed up. Heels about two inches apart.
2. Grasp both your hands firmly just below right knee and pull towards chest. Keep lower back flat against mat while performing exercise.
3. Repeat with other leg.
4. Now do this exercise by grasping both knees and pulling toward chest. Be sure your lower back is firmly against mat.
5. Hold to a slow count of three.
6. Work up to ten times daily.

Lumbar Exercise 1

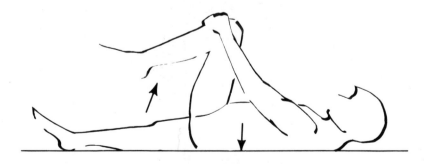

Figure 22

LUMBAR EXERCISE 2

1. Stand against wall, with heels as close to wall as possible.
2. Bend forward from the waist. Keep knees stiff. Exhale as you bend forward. Now slowly roll your lower back against the wall until you are erect. Be sure that all parts of the back are firmly in contact with the wall.
3. Tighten buttocks. It is important that the buttocks are tightened as you are rolling your back up the wall. Inhale as you roll your lower back against the wall and also draw in the stomach.
4. Relax.
5. This exercise can be done lying down on the floor if you are not able to do it standing up against the wall.
6. Hold to a slow count of three.
7. Work up to ten times daily.

A competency should be achieved in this exercise so that eventually you can press the small of the back against the wall by simply drawing in the stomach and tightening the buttocks.

Lumbar Exercise 2

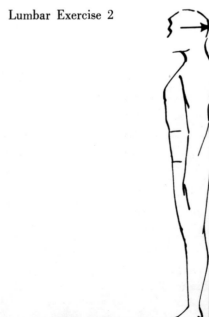

Figure 23

7. Scoliosis

SCOLIOSIS is the technical name for a sideways curvature of the spine. Most frequently there is no one specific cause for this condition although it may be caused by poor posture or perhaps by some body malfunction. At the outset it should be said that no one should attempt to deal with this disorder without help from a physician since its treatment is a strictly medical problem. However, it is certainly wise for everyone to be aware of this condition and its effects. A sideways curve also causes a loss in height. The amount of loss of course would be based on the degree of curvature. When scoliosis is corrected by surgery some patients may gain as much as two inches in height. We might mention that females are more prone to the sideways curvature than males. Also, the sideways curve can be divided into two categories—functional and structural. When we say that the curve is functional we mean that the curve will straighten itself out when we bend forward. If the curve does not straighten itself out then it is structural. See figure 24.

Generally, the sideways curve manifests itself most prominently during early adolescence. Early professional attention should be given to this condition since it may develop from a functional to a permanent type problem which might necessitate surgery. A sideways curvature could cause lung, heart or other body problems. The earlier one takes care of any body disorders, the better the chances are of achieving a cure.

Today, fortunately, scoliosis is being detected in school children by periodic physical examinations. Early detection makes it easier to correct.

Scoliosis

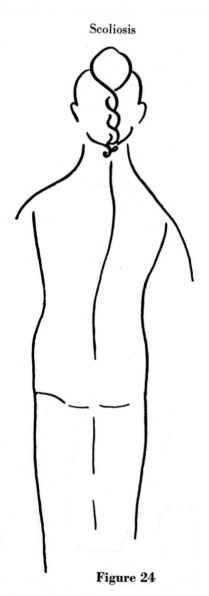

Figure 24

8. Knees

Knock-Knees

KNOCK-knees may occur at any age level but, unlike bowlegs, it is unusual to find it in infants. One or both legs may be affected. If a leg is broken or a knee injured and it does not heal

Knock-Knees   Knock-Knees Corrected

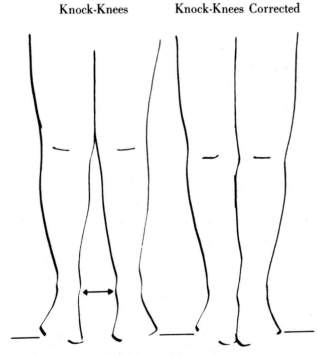

Figure 25

properly, a knock-knee condition may result. More frequently, knock-knees are directly related to such conditions as weak ligaments, poor arches and poor posture. The individual troubled with knock-knees, besides presenting a poor appearance, will tire easily and find it difficult to participate in sports. (See figure 25.)

To correct a knock-knee condition, a thorough examination is required. A physician commonly examines a patient and determines the degree of deformity by placing his hand or tape measure between the ankle bones. All aspects of the patient's condition which bear upon the deformity must be checked.

The importance of correcting knock-knees early is important. A slight case of knock-knees will tend to weaken the ligaments and, eventually, the arches and cause an altered weight distribution which in turn will increase the original deformity.

Bowlegs

It seems strange that what may be thought of as a deformity later in life occurs as a natural part of the growth pattern in early life. Bowlegs, for example, occurs quite naturally in children and is not a condition that parents should fret about. It corrects itself as the child grows older. Parents sometimes do a disservice to a child by forcing him to walk before the muscular structure is capable of supporting the youngster. This may then aggravate the bowleg condition which would prevent nature from correcting the condition naturally. Corrective treatment may then be necessary. Other situations which may aggravate bowlegs are sleeping positions, diapers and poor nutrition. (See figure 26.)

Bowlegs, of course, can occur at any time of life but whenever it occurs a physician should be consulted to institute remedial measures.

The loss in height from bowlegs would depend on the amount of angulation, but height loss might be considered minor compared to the other physical impairment it would cause to looks and body function.

Note the increased height with the bowlegged condition corrected.

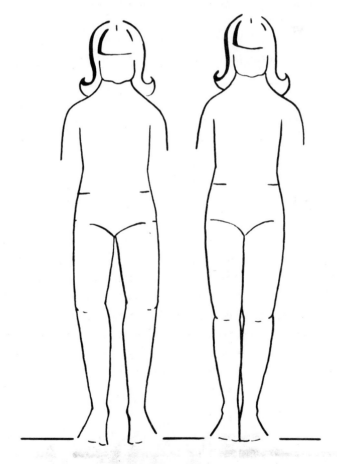

Figure 26

Knee Flexion

Knee flexion, or the bending at the knee, is a common postural defect which causes a loss in height and which is subject to correction. Technically speaking, we say that the knee is flexed when the angle between the two bones is decreased. (See figure 27.)

When we walk around with our knees constantly bent we create additional stress and strain on the muscles and ligaments. Of course when we have this additional strain we also become more fatigued as a result. Some individuals actually walk with their knee almost locked in the bent position. The following exercises are designed to correct this condition.

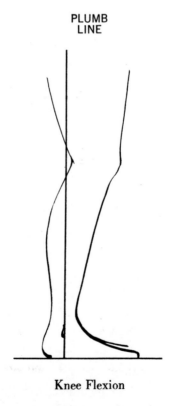

PLUMB
LINE

Knee Flexion

Figure 27

KNEE FLEXION EXERCISE 1

The following is a passive exercise:
1. Lie on abdomen on a firm surface.
2. Place rolled towel under leg just above knee cap.
3. Place approximately five pounds of weight on foot and suspend foot over edge of table.
4. Hold to a slow count of ten.
5. Remove weight and place foot in a comfortable position for twenty seconds.
6. Relax.
7. Repeat no more than five times.

Knee Flexion Passive

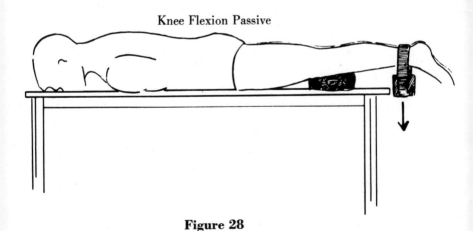

Figure 28

KNEE FLEXION EXERCISE 2

The following is an active exercise:

1. Sit with hips flexed at 90° angle as in figure 29.
2. Rest foot on stool with knee flexed at 45° angle as illustrated in figure 29.
3. Extend leg and straighten knee and hold to slow count of three.
4. As it becomes less difficult, gradually add weight on foot, up to five pounds.
5. Work up to ten times daily.

Knee Flexion Active

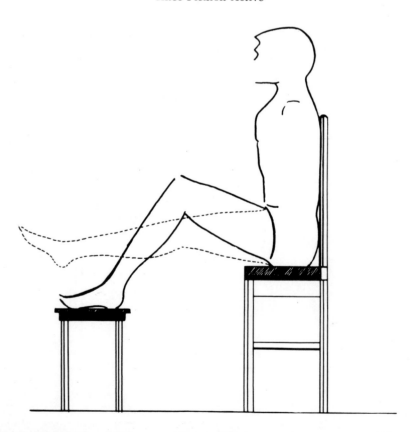

Figure 29

Knee Hyperextension or Back-Knees

Knee hyperextension is the opposite of knee flexion. In this condition (see figure 30) the angle between the bones is being increased. The back-knee condition will also cause a loss in height and in addition is usually connected with a host of other postural problems. Pain and overweight is also of significance with back-knee. Exercises for the back-knee problem will not be covered in this book.

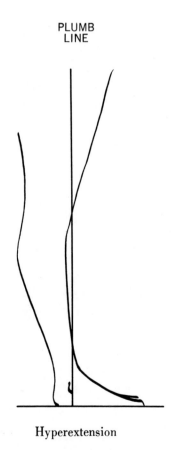

PLUMB
LINE

Hyperextension

Figure 30

9. The Foot

FEET are an important factor in posture and height. We will explore the problem in general, but it is well to remember that since so many difficulties of our body are interrelated, we separate and isolate them for purposes of organization. The pain in one's big toe, for example, may not be a toe problem at all, but a chemical one—that is, there is an excess of uric acid in the blood. And so we can say that the condition of one's feet may be due to a variety of causes ranging from heredity, diet, exercise, mode of living and type of footwear.

It is important to remember that exercise is vital in our daily life, but it is equally important to remember that the exercise must be the correct one. A proper exercise will do what it is designed to do but if it is used incorrectly, it can prove harmful. An individual might undertake foot exercises to correct flat feet but if this same person has a contracted calf muscle, the same exercises might aggravate the overall condition by further tightening the calf muscles.

Let us keep the lesson of Procrustes' bed in mind not only for exercises of the feet but for all body ailments. We will recall that Procrustes was a legendary figure who had an iron bed upon which he placed his victims. If the victim was too long, he cut him down to size; if he were too short, he stretched him to fit.

And so let us remember that we cannot give one overall prescription that will fit every individual even if the problem, let us say, of flat feet is the same. The cause for the flat feet may be different for each individual involved.

The normal foot is a sturdy and flexible mechanism which consists of twelve tarsal and metatarsal bones. The great toe contains two phalanges and the small toes contain three. Incidentally, the great toe carries one half of the body-weight, while the other toes carry the remaining half. (See figure 31.) The entire bony structure of the foot is stoutly held together by muscles, ligaments, and tendons. The entire grouping is intricately arranged to grip and move the body with great efficiency when it is functioning normally. But when it is faulty, we may then have a multiplicity of problems.

One of the most common problems is flat feet. Flat feet are generally due to stretched ligaments and poor muscles. We shall take this problem up a little later.

It is erroneous to think that one must wear shoes to support the flat feet or to wear arch supports and the like. You don't need arch supports any more than the normal person needs a

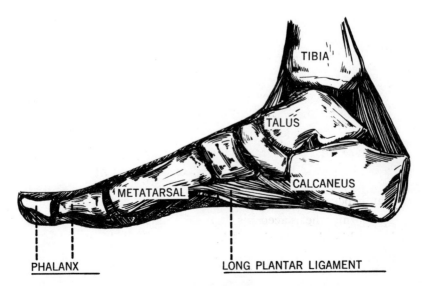

Figure 31

hearing aid. Wearing a brace when you don't need it only further weakens that which is being supported.

We should delve a little into the subject of shoes because so
much of our foot trouble today is due to shoes, despite the fact
that they were originally designed to protect the foot.

Mothers should be careful with their children with regard
to shoes. An infant is born with no arch but strong ligaments.
Sometimes parents try to show off the child and he is allowed
to stand for too long a time. If the child is overweight this may
result in overtiring the muscles and stretching the ligaments.
Let us remember that it is the ligaments and muscles that are
responsible for the arch.

For adults, be sure that the shoe is suitable for the occasion.
A shoe that is used for walking in the countryside should have
a thick sole and a sturdy toe cap. All shoes should be properly
fitted, not too large or too small and allowing at least ¼ to ½
inch room between the toe and the top of the shoe.

The adverse affect of high heels on the feet and our posture
is covered in another section of the book.

As we stressed before, the cause of a foot difficulty may not
lie in the foot. A complete examination by a physician is necessary to determine the possibilities of restoring the arch to a
flat foot. Therapy might include a wide variety of measures
from proper shoes, exercise, or even surgery. Please remember
that ligaments are not subject to voluntary control in the same
manner as a muscle. As far as the foot muscles are concerned
the most important one is the Tibialus posterior because it
curves under the horizontal longitudinal arch—it fans out and
gives general support.

One of the best exercises for the strengthening of the arch in
flat feet is walking around with bare feet and on tiptoe. This
should be done for about two hours in the evening. Children
and young adults are the most likely to benefit from this
exercise.

10. Poor Posture Habits

Models and Poor Posture

The next time you observe a fashion show, notice the postural positions assumed by the models. Perhaps the first thing you will notice will be the forward head. Closer observation will probably also reveal a faulty shoulder position, knees in a flexed or bent position and an exaggeration of the curve in the lower back. The abdomen will also be protruding. If continued this

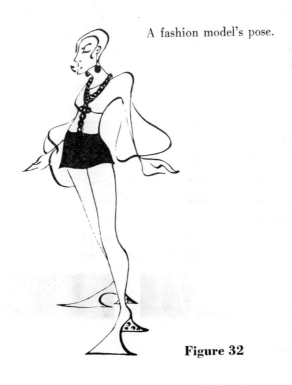

A fashion model's pose.

Figure 32

sort of position, if maintained for any length of time, may become a permanent part of an individual's stance.

As a matter of fact, you won't have to attend a fashion show to see the poor postural poses. Open up any fashion magazine and you will see a complete display of poor posture.

Figure 32 illustrates to a large extent what is wrong with our modern life in terms of posture. To some people, the exaggerated poses appear to be correct, yet every item, from the high heeled shoes she is wearing to the forward head position, is throwing the body out of its natural alignment.

How High Heels Shorten Your Height

It is appalling that so many people are unaware of the damaging effects of poor or improper footwear. We can certainly classify high heels on a shoe as improper. High heels, or even heel lifts, to increase your height will in fact produce the opposite effect. The chain of events that wearing high heels produces may extend from your big toe to your head.

Wearing high heels throws your hips or pelvis forward: When your pelvis is thrown forward, this accentuates or increases the curve in your lower back. It should be mentioned again that when we increase the curve in one part of the spine, eventually other parts of the spine must make a curve adjustment—and additional curvature results in a shorter spine and therefore lower height. (See figure 33.)

In addition to this the high heels flex or bend the knee and also shorten the Achilles Tendon (heel cord). Prolonged wearing of high heels may result in permanent shortening of the Achilles Tendon, a condition which may also produce low back pain and other body discomforts.

Some women after prolonged wearing of high heels are unable to walk properly in flat shoes or slippers—they must walk on their toes. It may even be necessary to lengthen the tendon by surgery.

High heels also prevent the ankle from being properly exercised, cause the calf muscles to tighten and contract, and the big toe to be hyperextended or turned up. The person wearing high heels takes shorter steps and, in general, his body takes on an unbalanced position. The sum of all these faults results in increased strain and tension. We must remember that when we have an unbalanced or faulty posture, this results in other parts of the body assuming new positions to compensate.

So, it is not being farfetched to say that the feet will affect the position of the head.

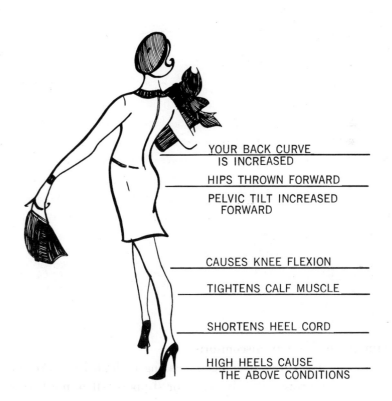

YOUR BACK CURVE
IS INCREASED

HIPS THROWN FORWARD

PELVIC TILT INCREASED
FORWARD

CAUSES KNEE FLEXION

TIGHTENS CALF MUSCLE

SHORTENS HEEL CORD

HIGH HEELS CAUSE
THE ABOVE CONDITIONS

Figure 33

The Knee Au Go Go

Of all areas of the body, the knee is one of the most vulnerable to injury. The knee connects the thigh bone or femur to the shinbone or tibia in a hinge-like arrangement. The femur or thigh bone, incidentally, is the biggest, longest and strongest bone in our body. The tibia or shinbone is the next strongest bone in our body and also a weight-bearing bone. A slender bone lying along the shinbone is called the fibula. It has no direct connection to the knee but is simply notched in at the end of the shinbone. The whole arrangement is firmly bonded by tendons, ligaments, cartilage, and muscle. Capping this joint is a protective piece called the knee cap or patella; for a lubricant in this mechanism we have synovial fluid. The patella or knee cap is attached by a tendon to a thigh muscle and to the lower leg.

The basic movement of the knee is bending. Now for the usual movements in life, the structural arrangement of the knee is perfect. Today, however, anyone who listens to the news or reads the newspaper is made aware of all the sports figures who are plagued with knee trouble. The knee was simply not designed to take the kind of punishment that is meted out in athletic contests.

The knee, wonderful mechanism that it is, cannot take the kind of jarring it is subjected to. Imagine a two hundred pound football player running down the field at full speed, suddenly slamming to a halt and then with equal vigor accelerating in a new direction—and *then* being pounced upon by other two hundred pounders. A stiff jolt in an encounter of this sort can be very damaging to the knee joint.

Dancing, for example, is wonderful for your posture and balance. (See figure 34.) And yet, today, we find an increasing number of go-go girls in the doctor's office complaining of knee trouble. Baseball, football, tennis and skiing, to mention just a few, have had their share of injuries. The thing to remember about a severe injury to the knee is—it's never the same again. More often than not, you will be plagued with this problem for the rest of your life.

Dancing can help posture.

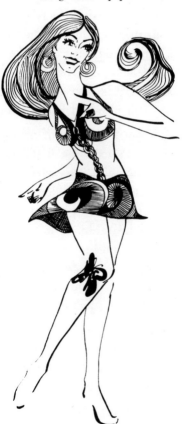

Figure 34

The Mattress, the Pillow, and You

We spend about a third of our life in bed sleeping or at least lying down. Movement, growth, and change continue even while we seemingly are not doing anything. Since this is the case, it behooves us to pay attention to what we are lying on. A saggy mattress with grooves that have been formed and shaped by some occupant over a long period of time is not conducive to good postural health. Once you slip into these grooves, free movement of the body is impeded. Depending also on how the mattress sags, one part of the body may be relaxing while another is under tension. The position may be such that breathing may be poor and your organs jammed into an uncomfortable or unnatural position. This could have, over the long run, harmful effects. It is a good idea to get a bed board for your mattress to firm it up. (A bed board is advised even if you have a brand new mattress.) A ⅝ inch plywood board is advised.

Many people ask about what kind of pillow they should use. Should one be used? Let's examine first what the pillow does to the head. There are actually three sleeping positions for the head. You can, for example, sleep face down on a pillow and if you have a large pillow this will bend your head backward— a position which is not desirable. Now let's say you lie flat on your back with your head on the same pillow: in this position your head is flexed or pitched forward. This position will give you a forward head which will throw your body alignment off and, over a period of time, can shorten your height.

Let us suppose you sleep on your side. In this position, your shoulder is actually propping your body up and, without a pillow, your head drops down. This is bad for your posture. A compromise must be made: a small pillow that will serve comfortably no matter what position you assume is the best choice.

Suppose you come home from work and you simply want to relax and rest. What is the best position to assume? See figure

35. A comfortable and relaxing postural position would be the following: place one pillow under your head and four pillows under your knees. In this position you will achieve relaxation of head, legs, and feet.

A comfortable, relaxing position.

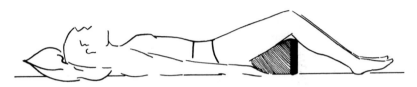

Figure 35

Sitting

Sitting is a postural position in which we spend a considerable amount of time. The same principles that apply to the standing posture are no less important in the sitting position. The back must still be properly supported and the pelvic girdle must assume the proper tilt.

It's unfortunate that human beings come in so many assorted sizes and shapes that finding chairs to fit everyone is a real problem. We shall soon see why. The chair must be of proper height. If the chair is too low you begin to slouch and thus put undue pressure on the lower back and the pelvic girdle. The length of the leg from heel to knee is the ideal height and from the back of the knee to the buttocks is the ideal depth of the seat of the chair.

Any variation from these dimensions will cause stress. Most manufacturers put out a standard size chair. The usual height of a chair is about 17½ inches. With the assorted sizes we have in the human family, not many will fit exactly into the mold that has been created. Ideally, everyone should have his own chair contoured especially for him. Children should have their own individual chairs. The assorted chairs, couches, sofas, and seats in cars, buses and airplanes are frequently poorly constructed and ill-shaped for lengthy sitting. It is no wonder the world abounds in so many back aches.

Let us not forget that there is an aesthetic and social value to proper sitting. We all want to make a proper appearance. People observe us as we sit, just as much as when we stand or stroll in our bathing suits on the beach. You are constantly making some kind of impression, no matter what postural position you are in. Figures 36 and 37 show proper and improper sitting positions.

Improper Sitting Position

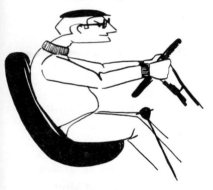

Figure 36

Proper Sitting Position

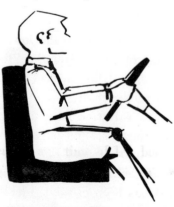

Figure 37

When the lower back is slumped and the head is thrust forward, we create conditions that unduly fatigue the body. Is it any wonder that an otherwise pleasant automobile ride ends up with an aching back and sharp pains across the shoulder area.

Hazardous Posture Positions

In the course of a day's activities, we are forced to take a variety of postural positions, some of which may be harmful if maintained for any length of time. The best policy, then, is to keep changing one's position so that no one postural stance is assumed for any length of time or any one group of muscles is overworked.

The way a student carries his books or how he studies at his desk could create a sideways curve of the spine. However, this may not be harmful or create any permanent damage if the student moves about and changes his position. Figure 38 demonstrates a type of activity that would curve the spine. Anyone

Some occupations produce additional strains on posture.

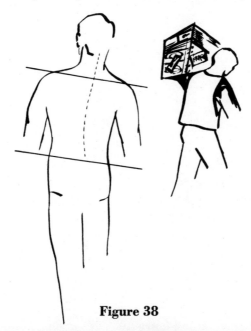

Figure 38

who engages in work which requires him to carry boxes or bundles on his shoulder should keep changing the load to the other shoulder periodically.

We should also be careful how we bend our body or how we push or lift an object. Some general principles that we should observe are: maintain a wide enough base to give your body stability when you lift a heavy object from the floor—that means spreading your legs and putting one foot ahead of the other. Bend your knees slightly. Keep whatever you are carrying as close to your body as possible. The further the load is from the center of gravity, the more instability we get. Don't let your lower back do all the work. Give those strong leg muscles a chance to get a workout.

We don't always have to get into some outlandish position to suffer a back strain. Sometimes this may occur (see figure 39) when we bend the upper trunk to brush our teeth or shave. So caution in our daily activities should be the watchword.

Improper standing position; knees should bend slightly.

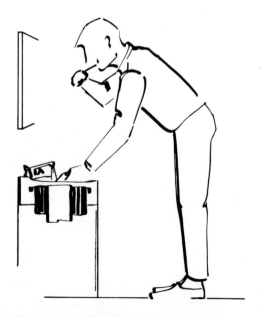

Figure 39

11. Glands, Hormones and Growth

As soon as a child is born the parents, relatives and friends are quick to remark on the appearance and general behavior of the youngster. Happily, in most instances, the remarks are complimentary and reassuring, and the proud parents glow with appreciation. With the passage of time, a watchful eye is kept on the child. Regular visits to a physician will enable the parents to double check their own observations. And there are guidelines that every parent should be aware of. The Human Growth Foundation has provided the following yardstick.

Does Your Child Measure Up?

America's kids come in all shapes and sizes. Many of the very short ones are going to be short or average sized adults. Some have serious growth disturbances which will keep them from reaching normal size. Answer the following questions about your child:

1. Is he the shortest in his class?
2. Is he still wearing last year's clothes?
3. When at play, is he unable to keep up with the other kids his age?
4. *Is he growing less than 2 inches per year?*

If you had four "yes" answers, you should suspect a growth problem and consult your physician. If he sees your child regularly, he can tell whether there is reason for concern. If there is a problem, he will evaluate your child or refer him to a doctor who specializes in gland and growth disturbances.

Most children with growth problems, apart from their size, are as normal as any other child. Some of their growth disturbances can be helped; some types will correct themselves in time. There are other types of growth problems for which medical research has not as yet found the answers.

Before we review how our glandular and hormonal system works, let us review some real life situations involving problems of growth.

Karen stopped growing when she was eight years old. She was just four feet tall. By the age of eleven she was so obviously smaller than her classmates and friends that she felt different and unhappy. Her parents, deeply concerned, brought her to North Shore University Hospital's Endocrine-Metabolism Ambulatory Program, Manhasset, New York, where it was found that her thyroid gland was inflamed and could no longer manufacture one of the hormones necessary for continued growth. Karen is now receiving daily thyroid hormone tablets and is growing at the rate of four inches per year. She can anticipate reaching her normal height, with no further problems.

Vital to Karen's "success story" is the fact that treatment was begun early, according to Fima Lifshizt, M.D., Pediatric Endocrinologist who is in charge of the Program. Later the damage would have been irreversible.

Hypothyroidism is only one of the growth problems which are cared for in the program. Sally had grown less than two inches since she was three years old, and at the age of five was only 30 inches tall. Her father built a special ladder so she could reach the bathroom sink. Her classmates in kindergarten carried her like a baby, although she was above average intelligence and could already read and write.

Sally was normal in all respects except for her size. On the advice of the pediatric endocrinologist she was admitted to a hospital where urine and blood tests revealed that she lacked the pituitary hormone which stimulates growth. With daily growth hormone shots Sally has grown over ten and one-half inches in the past three years.

Unfortunately all short statured children cannot be treated with growth hormones. However, they can be helped by psychological back-up to assist them in coping with their emotional problems, and by the acceptance and understanding attitudes of others. Short people are often treated with the thoughtlessness and ridicule that have marked them since the days of the court jester and Tom Thumb.

Short children may be perfectly proportioned or (as in achondroplasia) have small limbs, average size trunks, and large heads. In either case they face problems of adjustment to the physical environment—the first step on a bus, a light switch, the water faucet, a drinking fountain, and innumerable other objects present insurmountable obstacles.

Some children are "slow growers" who eventually attain a normal adult height, at times becoming even taller than many of their peers, but the spurt in growth and sexual development is late. This is usually familial and occurs frequently. There are no organic abnormalities; however, because it is so important in our culture to mature "on time" the young person needs reassurance to avoid adverse psychological reactions. At times treatment is indicated under the careful guidance of a pediatric endocrinologist. Inappropriate use of hormones could result in acceleration of growth for a shorter period with decreased eventual adult height.

Dr. Lifshitz stresses the importance of early and accurate diagnosis so that growth problems may be corrected if possible. Any disease in children may alter the normal growth

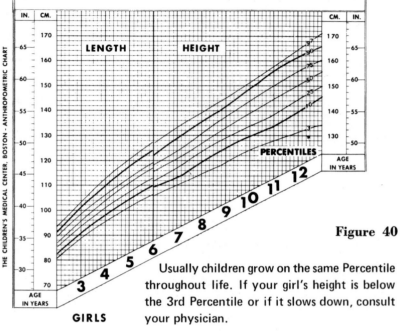

Figure 40

Usually children grow on the same Percentile throughout life. If your girl's height is below the 3rd Percentile or if it slows down, consult your physician.

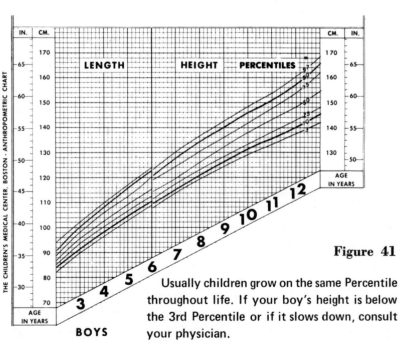

Figure 41

Usually children grow on the same Percentile throughout life. If your boy's height is below the 3rd Percentile or if it slows down, consult your physician.

process. Chronic infection, renal disease, and numerous other conditions must be ruled out. Counseling and guidance are available for the child who will remain small and must learn to make a place for himself in society. A positive self-image can help him withstand ridicule and the sympathy of well-meaning people who treat him as a child regardless of his age or intellectual level. Parents can also receive emotional support in handling the situation so that the child's best interests can be served.

History of Dwarfism

Dwarfism has been described since the Egyptian, Greek, and Roman eras. Dwarfs have entertained and served many monarchs as court jesters. The most famous American dwarf was Charles Stratton (nicknamed General Tom Thumb) of Bridgeport, Connecticut, who was 31 inches tall and who married Miss Lavinia Warren who was his size.

In 1908, the relationship between pituitary gland dysfunction and one type of dwarfism was recognized. Between 1908 and 1958 there was much scientific controversy as to whether humans required growth hormone for growth. Animal growth hormones were shown to have no biological activity in humans, although they stimulated linear growth at an extraordinary rate in animals that had had the pituitary gland inactivated. In 1956, the species specificity of growth hormone was recognized. In 1958, two groups of scientists receiving grant support from the National Institute of Arthritis and Metabolic Diseases (NIAMD) of the National Institute of Health, Bethesda, Maryland, extracted and purified a biologically active growth principle from the human pituitary gland which was called Human Growth Hormone (HGH) or Human Somatotropin. Under the impetus of this discovery, a whole new era of endocrinology has developed.

In the last 10 years, in contrast to the last 30 centuries, basic and clinical research has progressed rapidly in all areas of human pituitary physiology involving human growth hormone (HGH), human follicle stimulating hormone (HFSH), human luteinizing hormone (HLH), human adrenocorticotropic hormone (HACTH), and human thyroid stimulating hormone (HTSH). Clinical research has demonstrated the potential of HGH in the treatment of hypopituitary dwarfism and of human pituitary gonadotropins for the study of certain types of female infertility. New techniques have been developed for measurement of all these pituitary hormones in the minute concentrations present in circulating biological fluids. Rapid progress has been and will be made in the understanding of human endocrine physiology. The National Institute of Arthritis and Metabolic Diseases (with the cooperation of the College of American Pathologists) has been responsible for much of this progress through its grant support for both basic and clinical research and its contract support of the National Pituitary Agency.

Who Is a Dwarf?

By definition a dwarf is any adult 5 feet tall or less. Some may be as short as 18 inches. The words midget and dwarf are often erroneously used interchangeably to describe any adult of abnormally short stature. Midget correctly refers only to dwarfs with proper portions, i.e. all parts of their bodies are proportionately small. Unlike midgets, some dwarfs are abnormally proportioned with normal sized heads and trunks but with extremely short arms and legs. Dwarfism is a physical characteristic and has little or no effect on mental ability and development.

What Causes Dwarfism?

There are hundreds of causes of dwarfism—disease, improper nutrition, glandular disorders, hormone failure, and inherited short stature just to name a few. All the causes of slow growth are too voluminous to deal with here but some of the more common types are listed below.

Chromosomal Disorders

The most common chromosomal disorder is called the Turner's syndrome which is found only in girls. While scientists have been able to identify the chromosome abnormality they have not yet discovered its cause nor its cure. Girls with Turner's syndrome rarely grow to 5 feet tall and do not develop normal sexual characteristics.

Inherited Short Stature

Short parents tend to produce short children making genetic short stature the most prevalent of all types of dwarfism in the United States. Scientists are currently experimenting with human growth hormone (HGH) injections to help these children grow taller. Without help, some may grow no taller than 5 feet but will be normal in all other development.

Delayed Puberty

Normal adolescents experience a spurt of growth during puberty but some have a delayed puberty of 2 to 6 years. By the time they experience puberty their bone structure is too mature to react to a growth spurt and many of these children remain short. This delay is often inherited from one or both parents.

Bone Diseases

A recent scientific paper listed over 100 distinct bone diseases associated with short stature. Their medical names are usually tongue-twisters like achondroplasia, fibrous dysplasia, hypophosphatasia, mucopolysaccharidoses, osteogenesis imperfecta, etc. They result in deformed, shortened, or otherwise abnormally developed bones for thousands of children. One of the most common of these is achondroplasia which is characterized by a pronounced shortness of the arms and legs while the head is frequently large and the trunk normal size.

Primary Growth Disturbances

Children with primary growth disturbances seem to have body cells that do not respond to the usual growth-promoting factors. They have small proportional bodies and some have associated malformations of the head, ears, skin, brain, or one side of the body. One example is intrauterine growth retardation.

Secondary Growth Failure

Serious disease and strong drugs used in the treatment of disease may stunt growth. The disease or drugs may disturb bodily functions and produce an imbalance severe enough to slow down growth. Loss of appetite, damage to vital organs, vitamin and mineral imbalance, etc., can all result in poor growth and can all be caused by disease or drugs.

Hormone Failure

Growth is controlled by hormones produced by the pituitary gland. An organ about the size of a pea, the pituitary must produce enough human growth hormone (HGH) to affect normal growth. When it does not, hypopituitary dwarfism occurs. An adult hypopituitary dwarf may look like a child of 10 and usually has arrested sexual development. However, intellectual development, as in the case of most types of dwarfism, will be normal.

Nutritional Short Stature

Chronic malnutrition will prevent children from reaching their full genetic growth potential. Most common among these are children with a protein deficiency. If a child remains protein starved until the age of 5, the growth damage will be permanent.

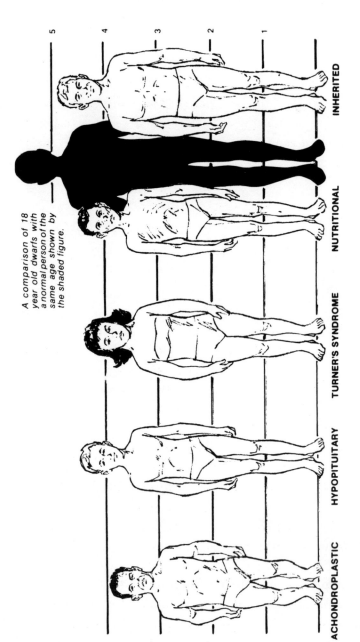

A comparison of 18 year old dwarfs with a normal person of the same age shown by the shaded figure.

ACHONDROPLASTIC HYPOPITUITARY TURNER'S SYNDROME NUTRITIONAL INHERITED

Figure 42

Can Dwarfism Be Cured?

Until recently little attention has been paid to the causes and cures of dwarfism. Research now is being conducted in all types of growth problems. With an estimated 500,000 children in the United States suffering from growth problems, this research is extremely important and long overdue.

One of the first breakthroughs in growth research was the discovery that human growth hormone could be extracted from the pituitary gland and injected into hypopituitary dwarfs to induce growth. Since 1963, HGH has been used in tightly controlled research projects to stimulate growth in over 500 dwarfed children. HGH promises to be a solution to hypopituitary dwarfism and a possible help to some other causes of dwarfism. Unfortunately, the supply of HGH depends directly on the donations of human pituitary glands—animal glands are not usable. Each child on the program needs from 50 to 200 pituitaries per year and the annual pituitary donations are only enough to accommodate a very limited number of children. Most of the children suffering from hypopituitary dwarfism cannot receive HGH treatments because there simply aren't enough pituitary gland donations to cover the need.

Synthesized hormone may be the next step in solving this problem. In early 1971, HGH was synthesized for the first time. It will take many more years to discover how to produce the synthesized hormone in quantities large enough to help the many dwarfed children who need it. And for some, it will be too late. Once a child's growth years end (usually between 17 and 21) HGH can no longer stimulate further growth.

Is Dwarfism Really a Handicap?

To some, it isn't. The pygmies of central Africa, the Negritos of the Philippines and New Guinea and the natives of the Andaman Islands in the Indian Ocean have been dwarfs for centuries. But in the American culture where the average male height is 5 feet 10 inches dwarfism presents a very real problem.

First, there is the physical problem of being too small to reach ordinary things like pay telephones, drinking fountains, mail boxes, wash bowls, door handles, elevator buttons, and so much more. Then there is the problem of being too small to participate in normal activities like sports, dancing, bicycling, driving, etc. Then there is the exceptional difficulty in shopping, finding a job, leading a "normal" life in a world too large for some little people to handle.

Most tragically, there is a psychological problem that all dwarfs must learn to handle. The jeers of classmates, the stares from adults, the jokes, the teasing, the loneliness of being "different" all present serious problems to dwarfs. Many overcome them with the support of well-informed, loving parents and friends. Others are not so fortunate and add life-long psychological problems to their already handicapped bodies.

We have examined the problems of growth. Let us now review in general how the body gland and hormone system works. A gland is a cell or a group of cells that manufactures secretions. There are two types of glands. One type has a duct. These are called exocrine glands. Our tear glands and digestive glands, for example, have ducts that introduce their secretions directly into a specific area. The other is a ductless gland. These are called endocrine glands. The ductless glands produce hormones that are introduced into the general bloodstream. Hormones do their work but are not changed. The word hormone comes from the Greek meaning to excite.

GLAND	HORMONE	WHAT IT DOES
Adrenals	Adrenalin	Raises blood pressure, heart and circulatory stimulant
	Cortisone	Controls salt balance and regulates body metabolism plus other functions
Islet of Langerhans	Insulin Glucagon	Sugar control Increases amount of sugar
Thyroid	Thyroxine	Controls body metabolism, affects the nervous system and influences growth
Parathyroids	Parathormone	Maintains calcium and phosphorous balance
Pituitary	Ten hormones, one of which is HGH (Human Growth Hormone)	Controls growth, stimulates sex glands plus a variety of other activities
Testes and Ovaries	Testosterone (testes) Estrogen and progesterone (ovaries)	Produces sex changes and changes in body development

Figure 43

There are six glands that produce hormones. They are adrenals, islet of Langerhans, thyroid, parathyroids, pituitary, testes, and ovaries. Figure 44 shows where these glands are located in our body.

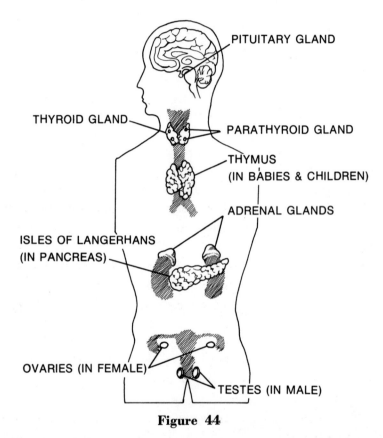

PITUITARY GLAND

THYROID GLAND

PARATHYROID GLAND

THYMUS
(IN BABIES & CHILDREN)

ADRENAL GLANDS

ISLES OF LANGERHANS
(IN PANCREAS)

OVARIES (IN FEMALE)

TESTES (IN MALE)

Figure 44

Figure 43 also indicates the name of the gland, the hormone that it produces and what it does. It is impossible in this book to go into all the details involving glands. From the previous material you have read, you can see the dramatic difference even a slight malfunction of glands will have on the body. Our body is in a constant state of dynamic balance. Underactivity or overactivity will have its countereffect in another part.

12. Nutrition

RECORDS are constantly being broken. For a long time, running the mile in less than four minutes was thought of as an almost impossible feat. And then on May 6, 1954, Roger Bannister, an English medical student, astounded the world by running the mile in 3:59.4 minutes. And then, hardly more than a month later, this mark was again broken by John Landy of Australia who ran the mile in 3.58 minutes.

And so we find that records are constantly being broken and new standards established. This same principle holds true for the human body with regard to the stresses, strains, and changes that it may be subjected to.

You may have noticed on a visit to a museum how man has changed in stature and build over the years. You probably observed that the medieval suits of armor were small and would never fit the average man of today.

Our height has been increasing over the years and these changes have been well documented. The U.S. Army measured a half million soldiers during the years 1863-1864 and their height averaged 67.7 inches. It's interesting to note that members of the U.S. Senate in 1866 averaged 69.5 inches in height —a difference of 1.8 inches. Why the difference? Studies that have recently been made show that groups that are economically more favored are taller than those not so favored. Studies that have been made in the United States and in Great Britain show that children from poor homes are two inches or more shorter than those from homes of the affluent. There is no reason to suppose that this was not the case back in 1866. U.S. Senators generally come from an economically favored group.

We again have Army measurements from 1917-1918. More than a million soldiers were measured and this time the height averaged 67.5 inches. This is a decrease in height and it is attributed to the fact that so many soldiers were immigrants or first generation Americans who were not as tall as Americans who had lived in the U.S. over a longer period. In 1946, 85,000 recruits were measured and their average height was 68.4 inches.

A life insurance study was made in 1912 of men thirty to thirty-five years of age. Their height averaged 67.6 inches. In 1955, a Department of Agriculture study of men aged twenty-five to twenty-nine showed an average height of 69.6 inches— an increase of two inches. Other studies also have been made of men at two colleges which reveal that freshmen in 1957 were three inches taller than freshmen in 1882. Also interesting is that height in certain categories increased. Only five percent of the freshmen in the 1880's were six feet tall. In 1955 about thirty percent of the freshmen were six feet or more.

And women cannot be left out of the picture. They also are growing taller. In the years 1900-1908 women twenty to twenty-nine years old averaged 62.4 inches in height; in 1955 they averaged 64.3 inches. Also, in 1900-1908, only a small minority (four percent to be exact) of women twenty to twenty-nine could be considered tall (at least 67 inches); in 1955, eighteen percent of the women were 67 inches tall.

That we have grown taller as a nation appears certain. But to what fact and circumstance can we attribute this? Good nutrition, better economic conditions, and better medical facilities seems to be the reason. Is there any special value in being taller? Being taller and being in better physical condition generally appear to be directly related to being better nourished. When we are well nourished and healthy, we are more productive, energetic, and creative. We thus can enjoy life more and contribute more to the life of the nation.

An interesting study was made by Lord John Boyd-Orr on the health of the Masai and Akikiyu tribes in Africa. Both tribes lived in the same general area. The Akikiyu lived on a high carbohydrate diet—fruit, roots, and cereals. The Masai tribe had a high protein diet—raw blood, meat, and milk. The mature Masai male was five inches taller and twenty pounds heavier than the Akikiyu.

Studies of Japanese children raised in the United States show that they are taller than their counterparts in Japan. Again this appears to be due to better nutrition. There can be little doubt that a nutritionally sound diet is essential if man is to achieve the full measure of health and stature that nature intended.

When we look at statistics from various countries around the world we find remarkable height increases over the years. England, Denmark, France, and Japan all report increases. Dr. Helen S. Mitchel, who studied nutritional problems in Japan, gave us the benefit of her observations in a very interesting report in the *Journal of American Dietetic Association.* For example, we generally think of the Mongolian people as being shorter than Caucasians but Dr. Mitchel questions whether it is really heredity. She feels that nutrition may well be the more important factor. Observers are noting that the college student in Japan is taller than his counterpart of a few years back. Heredity hasn't changed but the nutrition of the students has improved. Dr. Mitchel has observed that the tall person is especially admired in Japanese art and drama. Height is also admired in the United States, where there are economic effects as well. Leland P. Deck, personnal director at the University of Pittsburgh, made a study of one hundred students who graduated in 1967. Here are his results: those who were 6 feet 2 inches in height received an income that was 12.4 percent more than those who were less than 6 feet tall. Those graduates who were under 6 feet indicated an average salary of $701 per month; 6 footers got $719 per month and men who were 6 feet 2 inches got $723 per month.

The remarkable height increases that have been observed in Japan are credited to better nutrition—specifically, to the increase in protein. Dr. Mitchel noted that in a ten year period the consumption of protein increased ten percent but there was almost a doubling of animal protein. Although we generally think of protein as being important in building tissue, research indicates it is also important in bone growth. Dr. Mitchel's article also mentioned that supplementing the diets of 11 to 12 year old youngsters of farm families with lysine (an amino acid) increased their weight and height. Research, she reports, indicates that a proper balance of amino acid in the body stimulates growth.

The same pattern of height increase due to better nutrition has been confirmed by other studies. Dr. Mary Brown Patton and Fern E. Hunt also reported on height increases of Ohio school children in the *Journal of American Dietetic Association.* Measurements were made of 710 Ohio school children in 1939 and of 2700 in 1951. Again, those that were measured in 1951 were taller, and their diets were superior. Similar results involving height increases due to better nutrition have been reported by I. Leitch and A. W. Boyne in *Nutrition Abstracts and Reviews.* Dramatic increases in height up to 5 inches were recorded in measurements of boys 15 years old in 1925 and then among boys 15 years old in 1957.

Also, a study reported by Ruth Blair, Ph.D., Lydia J. Roberts, Ph.D., and Marjorie Greider, S.M., in the *Journal of Pediatrics,* noted the improvement in height among children in an institution when their diet was supplemented with dairy products, eggs, whole grain cereals, and pineapple juice.

Research in nutrition and its effect on the human body is progressing steadily. What we may think of as perfect height and health today may be changed tomorrow by some new discovery. We may not only be able to grow taller because of good nutrition and economic conditions, but we should also be able to extend our productive and creative life over a greater period. Of course as more and more people eat properly, we can expect a leveling off in height increases.

The picture in figure 45 gives dramatic evidence of the effect that a single food item has on animal life. No amount of words could convey how nutrition affects all living creatures. From this starting point let us examine how important nutrition is to our height and health. Although our main idea is the stress on height, still when we consider the subject, we must criss-cross the entire range of human health and that which affects it. Good height is a by-product of good nutrition, good housing, good living habits. With this in mind, let us explore health and height, beginning with the prenatal period.

The mother's responsibility toward her child starts long before birth. Her own state of health, and habits that she may have adopted, could have a decisive affect on the child's health and future development. Diet, drugs, and smoking, for example,

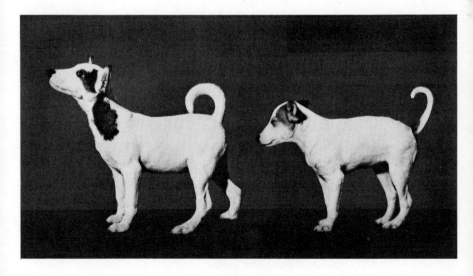

Figure 45

have a definite effect on the fetus, which will determine the infant's height, weight and overall health. The damage that has been caused to the fetus by drugs has been dramatically and tragically illustrated with the use of thalidomide by pregnant women.

Recent studies by Dr. Karlis Adamsons of Columbia University indicate that smoking is harmful to the fetus. Research indicates that infants born to mothers who smoke weigh less and are shorter than those who are born to non-smokers. The whole range of harmful effects remains to be studied. Other factors that may cause damage to the fetus are excessive x-rays, German measles, and drugs such as L.S.D.

We have evidence from experiments on animals on how nutrients effect living creatures. We can take risks and chances on mice, dogs, and monkeys that we would not dare on humans.

But sometimes events occur over which we have no control that enable us to make pertinent observations about nutrition and how it may change our growth and development. Such situations occur during wartime. Studies in Holland, during World War II, showed that women who had an inadequate diet bore children who were shorter and not as heavy as they would have been with a more adequate prenatal diet.

The same kind of results that were observed under wartime conditions have been confirmed by other studies. Bertha S. Burke, of the Harvard School of Public Health, found a definite statistical relationship between the diet of the mother and the weight and height of the children that were born.

A total of 216 women and their infants were involved in this study. Their diets were rated from good or excellent to poor or very poor. The women who were on excellent or good diets had the heaviest babies, the women on poor diets had the lightest babies. The same held true for height. The length of the babies was as follows:

Good or Excellent prenatal diet . . . . 20.393 inches
Fair prenatal diet . . . . 19.688 inches
Poor or Very Poor prenatal diet . . . . 18.582 inches

We cannot escape the conclusion that proper diet is vital for the mother and fetus. Moreover, evidence indicates it is the fetus that sustains the bulk of the damage when nutrition is inadequate in the mother.

If the child is off to a good start because of good prenatal nutrition, he has much to be thankful for. But a good start must be maintained. Adequate amounts of proteins, minerals, and vitamins must be supplied at all levels of growth. Inadequacies at any point create a poor nutritional jumping off place for the next spurt of growth.

And the young child does grow and develop rapidly. By the time he has reached one year of age he has tripled his weight and he is at least one-and-a-half times taller than at birth. After the first year growth slows down, the stage is now set for a somewhat different pattern of growth and development. At this point nature begins to put greater stress on the growth of the child's limbs in comparison to the trunk. At about a year-and-a-half the toddler's muscles begin to develop more rapidly. The reason for this can be readily seen: as the child now moves around more rapidly and has to support his body in a standing position, he needs the muscular wherewithal to do this. Also, his legs are pushing the body upward and moving the center of gravity away from his earth pad. The muscles involved are those of the thighs, buttocks, and back. Concomitant with the increasing muscular strength is the developing strength of the bones. Nature is slowing down the growth of the skeleton so that an increasing amount of minerals may be deposited. These minerals, especially calcium and phosphorus, are extremely important to maintain skeletal growth and to strengthen the bones. If youngsters between the ages of five and ten are deprived of adequate amounts of calcium, the growth of the skeleton may be retarded as much as three years. The absence of the proper minerals will cause growth to slow down and bones to become weak. If there is a serious deficiency rickets will develop. At any rate, we do not want any weakening or softening of the bone structure, since this could be the start of a postural defect and the cause of additional problems later in life.

The growth of muscle outpaces that of other tissue until the child is about ten, at which point muscle comprises about half of our body weight (the proportion that remains with us through adulthood). Of course we must remember that the youngster will need sufficient quantities of protein to keep building those muscles. That means plenty of milk, meat, and other foods that have an abundant supply of protein.

Milk is just about nature's most perfect food; there is really no substitute for it. It is an excellent source of high-quality protein, riboflavin, thiamin, vitamin A, vitamin B_{12}, and a superb source of calcium, which is so essential for bone formation. (The difference that milk made can be seen in the size and appearance of the two dogs in figure 40. The larger dog had an adequate diet of milk while the smaller one had none. Both dogs were from the same litter and, aside from their milk intake, their diet was the same.)

Maintaining proper nutrition is important at all age levels. Naturally, as we grow older there will be some variation in the amount and proportion of the various nutrients. We must remember that children from the age of one to the teen-age range need a greater amount of calories, proteins (the essential components of muscle and tissue), minerals, and vitamins in relation to body weight than adults. Children need the nutrients not only for growth and development but they must also store a certain amount. The best way to insure that a child has an adequate diet is to provide him with a wide variety of food.

Proper nutrition for the teen-ager should start in the morning with a good breakfast. This meal is so important, yet in too many cases it is eaten "on the run." You need a good breakfast to start the day in order to maintain the proper energy level for the morning's work (or school). A good breakfast would consist of proteins, such as eggs and milk; toast, jelly, and fruit would provide the balance of nutrients. This basic meal could be varied by consulting a good book on nutrition. Unfortunately, when a teen-ager misses breakfast, he does not usually make up for it at another meal. You must remember that breakfast should supply at least one fourth of the day's calorie and protein requirements.

Keep in mind that a child's rate of growth is uneven. The most rapid growth takes place within a period of two or three years, during which time proper nutrition is very important. While the adolescent is growing so rapidly, he should eat more than three meals a day in order to be supplied with all the nutrients his body will need—the proteins, the minerals and vitamins.

A look at the chart in figure 41 shows quite clearly how the growth rate of boys differs from girls. The girls outpace the boys and are generally taller than the boys in the twelve to fourteen age range. However, by the age of fifteen, the average stature of a boy is greater than a girl's.

The United States Dept. of Agriculture's Yearbook, *Food,* states that boys thirteen to fifteen years of age who weigh 108 pounds use almost as many calories (3,100) as a twenty-five year old moderately active man, weighing 154 pounds, who uses 3,200 calories.

Since adolescence is also a period of great emotional and social stress, it is important that energy and food requirements are met. If the youngster is fatigued because he lacks the proper nutrients, a chain reaction may set in that would affect his social life, school work, and posture.

If a person has been properly nourished throughout his life, he is lucky. Sometimes the results of poor eating habits can be corrected, sometimes not. Although our body requirements change as we grow into adulthood, the necessity for vital nutrients does not. You still need those proteins, minerals, and vitamins. Your body framework has been erected but it still must be maintained. If it is not properly nourished, fatigue will set in which then could affect your posture.

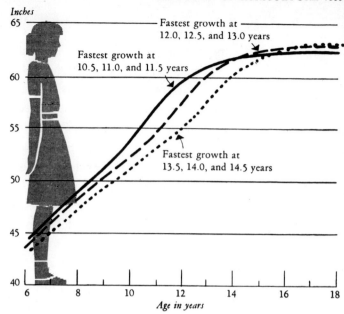

Average Heights of Girls Measured Yearly

Fastest growth at 12.0, 12.5, and 13.0 years

Fastest growth at 10.5, 11.0, and 11.5 years

Fastest growth at 13.5, 14.0, and 14.5 years

Inches

Age in years

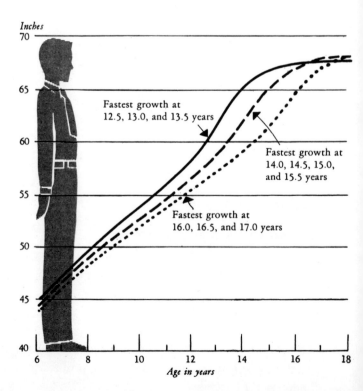

Average Heights of Boys Measured Yearly

Fastest growth at 12.5, 13.0, and 13.5 years

Fastest growth at 14.0, 14.5, 15.0, and 15.5 years

Fastest growth at 16.0, 16.5, and 17.0 years

Inches

Age in years

The Nutrients

Among the important nutrients that the body requires are the following: proteins, carbohydrates, and fats; minerals such as calcium and phosphorous; plus vitamins A, D, E, K, B, and C. An understanding of these nutrients is necessary if we are to know how our body functions and develops.

PROTEINS

Next to water, proteins constitute the largest portion of our body. With but a couple of exceptions, everything in our body contains protein. Blood, bone, teeth and muscle contain protein—even that tiny gene, so important in heredity, is composed of protein.

To illustrate the importance of protein, let's look at the results of an experiment conducted at the University of Nebraska with a group of 15 college girls. It was found that even when one glass of milk was eliminated from the breakfast meal it had an effect on the proper utilization of our food. (We will get more benefit from the proteins if they are distributed evenly among the three meals a day that we normally eat.)

The experiment at the University of Nebraska involved 15 volunteer college girls. The girls ate a nutritionally sound diet for 6 weeks with but one difference after the first 3 weeks. For the first 3 weeks the girls had one glass of milk with the noontime meal and 2 glasses with the evening meal. In the last 3 weeks of the experiment the glass of milk from the evening meal was added to the breakfast meal so that there was now one glass of milk for each of the meals. Everything else remained the same. The final results of this study showed that the proteins were more efficiently utilized when milk was provided with each meal.

Keep in mind that the following foods are good sources of protein; lean meat, fish, milk and milk products such as cheese, cottage cheese; also peanut butter, macaroni, plus a variety of vegetables. The vegetables vary in protein content, some are better sources than others.

CARBOHYDRATES

The rays of the sun in combination with air and a substance called chlorophyll are responsible for the carbohydrates that we eat. This is done by a process called photosynthesis. There is no other way that a plant can manufacture carbohydrates.

Carbohydrates, together with proteins and fats, form a nutrient group that provides man with energy. The carbohydrates can be broken down into three major categories—starches, sugars and cellulose. Starches are only a more complicated form of sugar. Cellulose, for all practicable purposes, is not digestable and passes through the body unchanged. However, it does serve the purpose of stimulating peristaltic action.

In the United States about half of our diet consists of carbohydrates; however, in other countries around the world the proportion is even higher. We in America happen to eat a great deal of protein, but other nations rely on cereals for nutrition. Cereals basically consist of carbohydrates, and are inexpensive, easy to grow and to transport.

Another benefit of carbohydrates is that they provide us with bulk and this is necessary to prevent constipation.

Carbohydrates in the form of sugar acts as a sweetener. We need carbohydrates to utilize or burn the fats properly. If the fats in our body are not burned or oxidized properly, we may accumulate what are known as ketone bodies and this may result in a disease called ketosis.

Carbohydrates also flavor our foods. There is such a thing as getting too much of a good thing but sweets can be used to entice youngsters to eat. The use of jam and jellies can be appropriate additions to our diet. Some foods perhaps have too much of an acid taste and only the addition of sugar makes them palatable. (Some foods nature sweetens herself to make them more palatable, such as young peas or corn.)

FATS

Today the word "fat" evokes a negative response from many people, and yet when we look at the situation from a historical point of view we find that this poor image did not always prevail. Fats at one time were treasured by people and were closely associated with prosperity and well being. However, because of the present association of fats and cholesteral with heart disease, this food element has come under closer public scrutiny. Their importance in our diet, therefore, cannot be disregarded.

Fats are made up of fatty acids in combination with other chemicals. The arrangement of the various fatty acids impart a definite characteristic to fats which will affect its nutritional quality. These fatty acids are essential to our diet and the full extent of how important some of them are has yet to be uncovered. Fats and fatty acids supply us with vitamins A, D, E and K and, in addition, they are the most concentrated sources of food energy—yielding 9.3 calories per gram. This compares to 4.0 calories for carbohydrates and 4.1 for protein.

It may be surprising to some people to note the many benefits that we get from fats. That fine flavor and satisfying taste in your food may very well be due to the fat content.

Furthermore, many organs of the body are supported, cushioned and protected by fat. Fat provides us with a reserve of food energy and it also provides passage for the fat soluble vitamins. In addition, it is a source of vital fatty acids which the body needs for growth and development. And remember on those chilly winter days that fats insulate and protect us from the cold. Also, fats, as is true of carbohydrates, conserve protein.

We cannot explore all of the fatty acids but certainly one of the most important is linoleic acid which is necessary for growth and for reproduction. Babies require it for growth and also to prevent skin problems. Breast-fed babies will have no problem since mother's milk is a good source of linoleic acid.

All of this does not mean that people must go out and purchase special nutrients to supply themselves with linoleic acid or any other nutrient. The average person will get all the nutrients he needs if he eats a normal diet.

THE VITAMINS

Vitamins play a vital role in our lives. We will discuss the specific effect of vitamins on our body and their importance. Although a certain nutrient may not directly impinge on growth and development, there is always the indirect effect that must be considered. Some vitamins are necessary for proper bone growth, others are necessary to protect us against infection. If our body has to spend time and energy to fight off infection, it then cannot develop properly in other aspects. We need good teeth, for example, to properly chew our food. It is not a farfetched assumption to assume that poor development in other areas of our body can also start as a result of poor teeth.

We classify vitamins by their solubility. Some, like vitamins A, D, E, and K, are soluble in fat and some, like C and B vitamins, are soluble in water. Stability and longer retention by the body are qualities that mark the fat soluble vitamins.

Vitamin A

Vitamin A is only present in animals. It is necessary for growth and specifically it is responsible for the quality of the outer layer of our skin and in keeping the mucous membranes and the digestive tract in a healthy condition. It is necessary to maintain proper vision, especially at night. Lack of vitamin A results in a condition known as night blindness. When we lack Vitamin A, the eye is not able to accommodate itself to seeing in the dark after exposure to light. It is also essential for the proper growth of bone and teeth, as well as for the protection against infections.

One way that our body obtains vitamin A is through a substance called carotene which is contained in yellow and green plants. Our body converts the carotene into vitamin A. The word carotene is derived from the word "carrot" since this is where it was first prepared from. When you see milk that is tinted yellow, it is due to carotene.

Green and yellow vegetables such as carrots, squash, sweet potatoes, pumpkin, turnip greens, kale, and yellow corn are sources of carotene; fruits such as apricots and yellow peaches are also good sources.

Valuable sources of vitamin A are the following: milk, butter, cheese, cod liver oil, and the egg yolks.

With vitamin A there should be this bit of caution: amounts in excess of what the body requires can result in hypervitaminosis.

Vitamin D

Vitamin D is essential for growth and development, especially of our skeletal structure and teeth. Without the proper amount of vitamin D, serious body ailments may develop.

Vitamin D was first isolated from cod liver oil in 1922. Previous to this, the curative power of cod liver oil for rickets was known, but the exact scientific reason was not determined.

Today, extreme cases of rickets are rare but in its milder

form it is still prevalent around the world. We can never become too complacent about any disease whenever there is a possibility of nutritional inadequacy. Rickets is a serious disease which can cause bowlegs, enlarged joints, and also defects in the rib cage, pelvis and skull. This poor body development can hinder your health and vitality for years to come.

Since vitamin D is so necessary for growth, and is not widely distributed in our food, scientists and health workers have been especially concerned that adequate amounts be supplied in our diet. Because milk is widely used—and also because it contains those other important nutrients, calcium and phosphorus—it was decided to fortify each quart with 400 units of vitamin D.

Good sources of vitamin D are cod liver oil, canned salmon, herring and mackerel. Dairy products, egg yolk and liver are also sources of vitamin D. Sunlight is another way of getting vitamin D; the ultraviolet rays acting upon our body create vitamin D.

As with vitamin A, there is a danger of being overdosed with vitamin D. Though we need vitamin D in sufficient quantities to maintain health, taking more than is necessary can lead to serious consequences.

Vitamin E

Vitamin E is an essential nutrient and its therapeutic benefits have been hailed by many as everything from an agent to protect the heart to a possible anti-aging substance.

Vitamin E was first discovered in 1922. Much of what we know about vitamin E has been due to experiments on rats. Although a good deal of the results and information that we have obtained is not applicable to man, they are, nevertheless, interesting.

When pregnant rats are on a diet that is deficient in vitamin E, they are unable to carry the fetus to full term. The usual time for the fetus to develop in a rat is about 21 days, but in the absence of vitamin E, the fetus begins to die soon after the fifth day of pregnancy. If vitamin E is administered at any time up to the fifth day, the mother can deliver a healthy rat.

With rats it is not only the reproductive process that is affected. Young rats that are deprived of vitamin E over a period of time lose vitality and fail to gain weight. There is also an overall growth slow down.

In human beings vitamin E has an important function as an antioxidant. This means that it is capable of combining with oxygen in such a manner that it protects the red blood cells from destruction.

Although many of you have already heard of vitamin E and its many possible uses, I'll wager that very few have heard of an ailment called Duprytren's Contracture. This condition occurs mostly in middle aged men and involves the fingers which contract. It was Baron Dupuytren, a French surgeon, who described the condition.

We will not go into all the technical aspects of the problem, but basically what is involved is this: The muscles and tendons force the fingers to contract and if the condition continues, only surgery can offer possible relief. However, if the condition is detected early enough, vitamin E has been reported to cause a regression of the disease. Once the ailment gets beyond the early stage, vitamin E is of no use. The vitamin E treatment has been known for over a quarter of a century. Unfortunately, in some cases even surgery does not help and the patient must keep his fingers contracted; he cannot extend his fingers and thus has only partial use of his hand.

Vitamin E is present in a wide variety of food-stuffs, but some of the best sources are lettuce and wheat germ oil.

Vitamin K

Vitamin K is primarily associated with the clotting ability of blood and the formation of prothrombin, a protein, by the liver.

When the body does not have sufficient vitamin K, it takes longer for blood to clot, thus increasing the chances of hemorrhaging. Vitamin K is contained in a wide variety of foods such as green leafy vegetables, egg yolk, and all types of liver.

Vitamins B and C

Vitamin B and vitamin C are known as the water-soluble vitamins; their ability to be stored in our body is very limited.

The seven members of the vitamin B group that are essential to human health are: thiamine (B_1), riboflavin (B_2), niacin, pyridoxine (B_6), pantothenic acid, folic acid, and vitamin B_{12}.

Thiamine (B_1)

The importance of thiamine may come into our minds when the word beriberi is mentioned or even the term, polished rice. Even as school children we learned that more than the outer skin of rice was lost when it was polished. Such polishing removes thiamine and other vital nutrients. Beriberi, a disease caused by thiamine deficiency, troubled the Japanese Navy for many years. The disease causes a wasting and weakening of body and nerve tissue. Even during World War II, the Japanese armed forces were troubled by vitamin B_1 deficiency. Soldiers ate polished rice which was deficient in thiamine and many of them were sidelined.

Our body needs thiamine to provide an energy releasing function in combination with other substances. It is also needed to promote normal growth. Because thiamine is not stored to any large extent in our body, we should have a daily supply. The recommended allowance per day is 0.5 milligrams per 1000 calories. One of the best sources of thiamine is lean pork. Other good sources are poultry, fish, milk, and eggs. The fact that bread and cereals are enriched is helpful in supplying thiamine. One of the unfortunate things about thiamine is that it is so unstable. Overheating and overcooking destroy sizeable amounts.

Extreme deficiency of thiamine will cause beriberi but a lesser deficiency will result in a loss of appetite and weight, fatigue, irritability, moodiness, and depression. (The fact that fatigue can affect posture has been discussed earlier in this book.)

Beriberi is rare in the United States but numerous individuals still suffer from a lack of thiamine. In this category would be the person who consumes alcohol to excess. Alcohol depletes the body of thiamine. In fact it would appear that even if a person were going out for an evening and anticipated drinking more than the usual amount, it would be wise to supplement the diet that day with extra vitamin B_1.

Riboflavin

The importance of riboflavin was recognized in the latter part of the nineteenth century but it wasn't until the early 1930's that its true significance was known. Continued research since then has disclosed that riboflavin acts in concert with protein to create enzymes which are needed for proper body functioning. Experiments with animals show that the lack of riboflavin affects growth and longevity. With human beings it may result in a disease called ariboflavinosis. This disease causes changes in the mucous membranes of the mouth and sores around the nose.

Good sources of riboflavin are milk and cheese, meat, especially liver, also eggs and various green leafy vegetables. Enriched bread and cereals are also valuable sources.

Niacin B₃

Niacin, as is true of thiamine and riboflavin, acts as an energy releasing agent in our body. It does this by working in partnership with enzymes. An enzyme is known as an organic catalyst that is formed by living cells. They speed up chemical change without being changed themselves.

Pellagra is a disease that has long been associated with a diet deficient in niacin. Pellagra is a disease that affects the body in various ways, including the nerves and digestive system. This disease was very prevalent in the South from the early 1900's till the late 1930's.

A researcher, Joseph Goldberger, discovered that certain protein-rich foods prevented or cured pellagra. Work continued on this problem and in 1937 Conrad Elvehjem of the University of Wisconsin fed nicotinic acid to dogs with black tongue, a disease comparable to pellagra in humans. Nicotinic acid cured the black tongue; nicotinic acid was added to the list of known vitamins and its name was changed to niacin to avoid confusion.

Since the discovery of niacin, its role in medical treatment has been expanding. Leading workers in the psychiatric use of niacin are Drs. Abram Hoffer and Humphry Osmond.

Niacin, depending on the dosage, will give a reaction—a flush, lasting for perhaps 20 minutes or more.

Many beneficial results have been reported for niacin—relief of allergies, emotional tension, headaches, and psychiatric problems. B_3 can also be taken as niacinamide. There is no flush when taken in this form. Anyone contemplating long-term therapy with B_3, especially in megadoses, should consult a physician.

Pyridoxine (B_6)

Vitamin B_6 is made up of a group of three chemicals, technically called pyridoxine, pyridoxal, and pyridoxamine. This vitamin is present in many foods, such as liver, various muscle meats, and a great variety of vegetables. Cereal grains, especially bran, is a notably good source.

Vitamin B_6 plays a role in a variety of body activities, some of which are still under investigation. Infants require it for proper body metabolism. Its need may become increased for pregnant women because of chemical changes that take place at this particular time.

Vitamin B_6 plays a part in the metabolism of tryptophan, an amino acid. Tryptophan is an amino acid that is essential for the nutrition of man.

Experimental deficiency of B_6 has been produced in adults. The resulting symptoms included depression, sleepiness, and a number of other uncomfortable body conditions.

It appears that women who are on "the pill" need an increased amount of vitamin B_6. The estrogen in "the pill" causes the body to use increased amounts of pyridoxine. The body is a very delicate chemical machine and when any undue disturbance occurs, it pays a price.

Many pregnant women who feel nauseous feel a sense of relief when they supplement their diet with extra vitamin B_6.

Pantothenic Acid

Pantothenic acid is essential to man. It is present in such a wide range of food products that it is highly unlikely that anyone would suffer from a shortage of this vitamin. It is present in liver, lean beef, kidney, potatoes, broccoli, tomatoes, skim milk, and whole grain cereals.

One of the ways we can find out how a vitamin affects people is to deprive them of it. When subjects were deprived of this vitamin by the use of a substance that closely resembles pantothenic acid, but didn't function like it, the following results were noted. They became sullen and quarrelsome, lost appetite, and developed indigestion and a variety of other physical disturbances.

Folic Acid

Folic acid is necessary for the production of red blood cells in our body. The exact role and its interaction with other substances in our body is under continuing investigation. We do know that Folacin can be synthesized by intestinal bacteria and this, very likely, is an important source. Current thinking is a regression of the disease. Once the ailment gets beyond the that about .5 milligrams per day should be sufficient. Certain drugs can produce deficiencies of folic acid.

For example, an individual suffering from Toxoplasmosis has a disease caused by the parasite T. Gondii. One possible problem of this disease is visual impairment. Now the therapy to kill the parasite involves using the drug Daraprim. Daraprim depletes the body of folic acid and this in turn makes the patient nauseous plus other possible side effects.

In order to overcome this condition the patient must be given injections of folinic acid. It must be given by injection because it cannot be properly absorbed by taking it orally.

Vitamin B_{12}

The lack of vitamin B_{12} is the cause of pernicious anemia in man. It isn't that vitamin B_{12} is not present in the diet, but it is a failure of the vitamin to be absorbed through the intestinal tract because of the absence of what is called the "intrinsic factor" in gastric juice. When this factor is not present, vitamin B_{12} cannot be absorbed into our body.

Until 1926 pernicious anemia was an incurable disease which in the United States alone caused thousands of deaths. Drs. George R. Minot and William Murphy discovered that victims of this disease could be treated by feeding them large amounts of liver. Later the liver became available as an injectable extract. These shots, however, were uncomfortable to patients.

Work to isolate the exact substance that would be effective against pernicious anemia continued. Finally, in 1948, Edward L. Rickles and his associates isolated B_{12}.

At about the same time, Lester Smith, in England, also isolated the vitamin. Randolph West of Columbia University demonstrated that B_{12} given by injection was effective in the treatment of pernicious anemia.

We are still learning about vitamin B_{12} and how it is involved in a wide range of bodily processes. It is essential to growth, cell reproduction and it appears to have a role in the function of nervous tissue.

One of the more interesting studies regarding B_{12} was conducted by Drs. Ellis and Nasser. They reported their findings in the *British Journal of Nutrition* (1973). It was a pilot study of B_{12} on the treatment of tiredness. The researchers had noted that previous investigators commented that B_{12} increased one's energy and improved the general well-being of patients.

Drs. Ellis and Nasser wanted to back up these claims with

a precise scientific study. Subjects were selected from volunteers and physician referrals. Careful physical exams were given to each volunteer to rule out medical causes of fatigue. The main complaint of those in the study was that they suffered from tiredness or fatigue.

The results of the test indicated that B_{12} by injection had a beneficial tonic affect. Just precisely how this vitamin works to give these favorable results is still subject to speculation.

Drs. Ellis and Nasser also mention in their study the role that B_{12} has in the treatment of tobacco amblyopia (reduced vision). Individuals who smoke have an excess of cyanide ions present in their body. B_{12} has an attraction for these cynanide particles and these individuals therefore benefit from this vitamin treatment.

Vitamin C

The value of vitamin C or Ascorbic acid to the human body has come into increasing prominence lately as a result of the work of a number of scientists. However, the writings and speeches of Dr. Linus Pauling, a Nobel prize winner and author of the book *Vitamin C and the Common Cold* has lurched the subject into a cauldron of hot activity. Positions for and against Dr. Pauling's views were hotly debated.

There was never any question that vitamin C is essential to human life. The debate centered on the quantity that was required on a daily basis and the quantities that may be required to stave off or cure various ailments.

Vitamin C has the least stability of all the water-soluble vitamins. It is very vulnerable to heat, light, and certain chemicals. Since it is water-soluble, large amounts of the vitamin can be lost in the water. Also, the capacity of the body to store vitamin C is very limited.

Although vitamin C, as such, was unknown many centuries ago, it was observed that fresh fruit could prevent scurvy, a disease that causes loss of energy, hemorrhaging, anemia, leg pains, and general weakness. When British sailors in the eighteenth century came down with scurvy, it was observed that fresh citrus fruit was an excellent preventive. And so it came to pass that lemons or limes became a stock item aboard British ships.

However, the nutritional importance of vitamin C ranges much further than the prevention of scurvy. Vitamin C is necessary for proper growth. The bones of infants will not grow properly if the supply is inadequate. Vitamin C is necessary for the assimilation of iron and also for proper cell maintainment. It also helps in combating infection and assists in the healing of wounds.

The history of vitamin C is certainly interesting. Charles King and a graduate student, William Wargh, isolated vitamin C from lemons in 1932. They identified it as the scurvy-preventing vitamin. Actually, Hungarian scientists had identified it four years earlier, but they were more interested in its other interesting chemical properties. The chemical structure of vitamin C is relatively simple and how it acts as a chemical is known.

Vitamin C occurs in animals, fruits, and vegetables. Most animals can manufacture their own vitamin C. Only humans, monkeys, and guinea pigs must get it from sources outside their own bodies. Humans, monkeys, and guinea pigs show the same signs of physical destruction when they are deprived of vitamin C.

Vitamin C or ascorbic acid is a specific chemical substance. Its chemical formula is as follows:

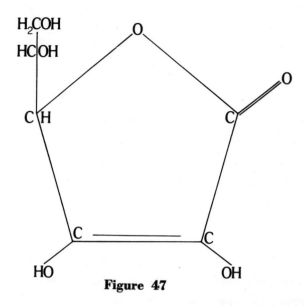

Figure 47

Ascorbic acid was the first vitamin to be prepared by total synthesis. This chemical is the same whether it comes from the orange juice you drink or is made synthetically in a laboratory.

If your body gets more ascorbic acid than it needs, it is then excreted from the body with the urine. How much vitamin C does our body need? Well, the evidence seems to indicate that as little as 10 to 20 milligrams of vitamin C will prevent one from contracting scurvy. But the evidence also shows that much larger amounts may be needed in some cases to really keep the body in tip-top shape.

Because of the connection between infection and vitamin C, higher doses of vitamin C are sometimes recommended. A lack of vitamin C carries the risk of infections. There is some reason to believe that the production of anti-bodies (disease-fighting mechanisms) is impaired if we do not have the proper supply of vitamin C.

People who smoke also have lower blood levels of vitamin C than nonsmokers, even though both groups consume the same amount of vitamin C.

MINERALS AND ELEMENTS

Calcium and Phosphorus

Calcium and phosphorus are the twin elements that provide the basic mortar for our bony skeleton. And, as we know from our previous discussions, faults in our basic skeletal structure and its alignment will affect our entire body.

Of our total body weight, four percent is composed of minerals, and better than half of this four percent is calcium and phosphorus. We find that 99 percent of the calcium and 80 to 90 percent of the phosphorus in our body is in our bones and teeth. The rest is distributed in the other body tissue and fluids.

In addition to providing building material for our bony structure, calcium is an essential agent in blood clotting, controlling and regulating the beat of the heart, enzyme activity, and nerve function.

Phosphorus is extremely important in cellular life, involved in a whole series of activities concerning body nutrients and in maintaining proper growth and stability of the body chemical system.

The case for calcium and phosphorus and the other nutrients involved in body building and their possible effect on height is very well stated in the *Yearbook of Agriculture:*

> The intricate process of bone building requires many nutrients besides calcium and phosphorus. Vitamin D is essential for absorption from the intestinal tract and the orderly deposition of the bone material. Protein is needed for the framework and for part of every cell and circulating fluid. Vitamin A aids in the deposition of the minerals. Vitamin C is required for the cementing material between the cells and the firmness of the walls of the blood vessels.
>
> Bones can accumulate a reserve supply of calcium and phosphorus at any age if the diet provides enough for the growth and repair and some is left over for storage.
>
> When the intake is generous, the minerals are stored inside the ends of the bones in long needlelike crystals, called trabeculae. This

reserve can be used in times of stress to meet the body's increased calcium needs if the food does not supply enough.

When there is no reserve to use, the calcium has to be taken from the bone structure itself—usually first from the spine and pelvic bones. The dentin and enamel of the teeth do not give up their calcium when the body must provide what the diet lacks.

If the calcium that is withdrawn in times of increased need is not replaced, the bone becomes deficient in calcium and subnormal in composition. From 10 to 40 percent of the normal amount of calcium may be withdrawn from mature bone before the deficiency will show on an X-ray film. Height may be reduced as much as 2 inches because of fractures of the vertebrae, which are caused by pressure and result in rounding of the back. Such fractures may occur with relatively minor jolts or twists of the body and may not be recognized at the time they happen.

Bones with a low content of calcium are weaker and break more easily than bones well stocked with calcium. Breaks in older persons often are related directly to the thinness and brittleness of the bones and are difficult to treat. The bones may be too weak to hold pins or other means of internal repair, and healing may be slow because of the low activity of bone-forming cells.

And the *Yearbook of Agriculture* has this comment which should be of interest:

Calcium appears to have an added function in the atomic age. It may reduce the amount of radioactive strontium 90 that may be deposited in the body.

Strontium 90 is a product of atomic explosions and may become a health problem. Its radioactivity is slow to disappear, and its accumulation in the body could be dangerous. Strontium 90 is absorbed into the body from the food and then deposited and retained in the bones. High concentrations of it can cause bone cancers and possibly leukemia, the blood cancer that begins in the bone marrow.

Major atomic explosions (described as megaton size) send the strontium 90 into the upper atmosphere and scatter it widely. When it returns to earth, it is deposited rather thinly on the soil and plant foliage over large areas.

The smaller atomic explosions (described as of kiloton size) do not send the strontium 90 up so far, and it is deposited more thickly on the soil and plants near the site of the explosion.

Strontium 90 was first detected in animal bones, dairy products, and soil in 1953. It now occurs in all human beings regardless of their age or where they live.

The lack of calcium can affect one's stature in a very direct way and also permanently damage the skeletal structure. It is wise, therefore, to see that one is not deprived of this important element—at any stage of his life.

Excellent sources of calcium are milk and milk products. Excellent sources of phosphorus are milk, meat, egg yolk, and fish.

Sodium and Potassium

We will deal with sodium and potassium as a single unit because they are so similar in their chemical properties. It is interesting to note how these two elements operate within our body. Potassium is within the individual body cell with very little outside the cells; sodium is present mostly outside the cell in the circulating fluids. Sodium and potassium are necessary to keep a proper balance of water between body cells and surrounding fluids. Both elements are essential for our nervous system to properly respond to various stimuli. Sodium and potassium work in conjunction to maintain the correct acid–alkali balance in our body. Various body muscles including the heart muscle are influenced by potassium and sodium. Individuals who take diuretics deplete their bodies of potassium and thus require additional amounts.

Sodium is an element that we are well supplied with. This oversupply occurs because we add it to our food. Some people add such amounts that they cannot taste the sodium which is present in the food naturally. People who normally salt celery cannot taste the natural salt in it. An individual who is careful about the amount of salt he uses can taste the natural salt in celery.

Magnesium

Magnesium is a white mineral element. Since it occurs in man in such large quantities we cannot really call it a trace mineral. There is a close relationship of magnesium to both calcium and phosphorus. We find that about 70 percent of the magnesium that we have in our body is in the bones. The remainder is located in the blood and soft tissue.

Magnesium is what we call a starter in a chemical action that our bodies must undertake. It is needed for the synthesis of protein and is involved in an entire array of body growth and maintenance. Also, it is important in the movement of potassium and sodium across the cell membranes. A deficiency of magnesium will disturb the calcification of bone. Animals that are deficient in magnesium become very nervous. The adult requirement of magnesium is about 0.3 grams a day. The body of an adult has about 21 grams of magnesium.

Magnesium in combination with other minerals helps maintain muscle balance and steady nerves. It also helps to keep the proper iron balance and osmotic pressure in the body.

Two of the body's major systems—the central nervous system and the cardiovascular system—can be affected by either an undersupply or an oversupply of magnesium. However, it is usually an undersupply that affects people the most. The technical name for an undersupply is called hypomagnesemia; an oversupply is called hypermagnesemia.

We sometimes become frightened when we see a long word, technical jargon so to speak, but if you look at a word and then break it down into smaller parts, it will not appear so overwhelming. *Hypo* is of Greek derivation meaning less than and *hyper*, also of Greek derivation, means above or excessive.

Let us go a little further regarding hypomagnesemia. Your

central nervous system may be affected with disturbances such as insomnia, muscle weakness, or leg or foot cramps. Your cardiovascular system may be affected by an irregularity of the pulse and a lowered blood pressure.

Manganese

Manganese is a metal element which is found in many plants and animals. When we talk about many of these trace elements we must remember that research as to their importance and their activity is still going on. Sometimes we think that growth is normal even if the constituent was not present in the diet. We really cannot use that sort of definition. Sometimes it is very difficult to determine if all our physiological processes are working in a perfect manner.

Manganese is essential for bone growth and tissue respiration, and, to many, it is necessary for the synthesis of ascorbic acid. Plus, it aids in many complex functions in the body.

Copper

Only small amounts of copper are needed by the body. It works in connection with iron to form hemoglobin. It is an aid to tissue respiration. Copper is present in the liver at all times. Excess copper is excreted by the liver.

Zinc

Zinc, in its natural state, is a white crystalline substance. Yet this metalic element in small quantities has a recognized function in the body's processes which is so essential to life.

A person should get at least 0.3 milligram per kilogram of body weight. A kilogram is equal to 2.2 pounds.

Zinc appears in our soil as a salt. Under heavy rainfall, for example, much of this salt may be washed away. Consequently, the food that is produced from this soil may be low in zinc. Also, when we cook our food we may be throwing away much of the zinc that is present. Studies indicate that zinc promotes the normal growth of people. Growth retardation may indicate a deficiency of zinc.

Iron

Iron is essential for the formation of hemoglobin in the blood. Iron combined with oxygen is absorbed by plant life. It carries oxygen which helps produce chlorophyl.

An adult body has about 3 grams of iron. Most of this is in the red corpuscles.

As essential as iron is to the body for tissue respiration and the development of blood cells we must also be aware of the hazards of too much iron. Damage to the liver, heart and other organs may result from an excess of iron.

Sulfur

Not many people think of sulfur, that yellow, crystalline element, as essential to life. This substance which burns in its pure form with a blue flame is a constituent of every cell in our body. Sulfur content is also high in our nails, hair, and bile. Eggs have a particularly high sulfur content. A deficiency of sulfur in our body may show up with imperfect development of nails, hair and various skin defects.

Iodine

Iodine is a trace element which has been used in medicine since the early nineteenth century. It is necessary for the proper functioning of the thyroid gland and to regulate the basal metabolism rate of our body. Growing children and those individuals who are under emotional strain need additional amounts of iodine.

13. Body Image

OUR body image consists of the total idea we have of our body —the way it appears to us and how we conceive of it appearing to others. The image we have started from the day we were born. One was not conscious of it, but everything that was happening around us had its impact.

Our parents exerted a tremendous influence. All the gentle acts of hugging, kissing, and fondling—all of the warmth and acceptance that a child is given—start the initial impetus toward the positive and strong image we will eventually have of ourselves.

The child who is ignored or left to himself for extended periods of time or not greeted with a true sense of love, is starting on a path that could have deep psychological and emotional impact which could prevent him from coping with life's problems in a sensible and adequate fashion. If the child grows up with a poor picture of himself, he is hardly in a position to judge those around him. It is like taking a picture with a camera. If all the adjustments for light and distance are not accurate, the picture we get will not correctly reflect the reality that we sought.

We must remember that even under the best of circumstances, the results that we may expect from a youngster may run far short of our expectations. Despite the best of intentions, things will go wrong. We do not have control of every aspect of the child. The inherited characteristics will not respond in the same way as those of another child, even in the same family.

We can take a perfectly stable family—mother, father, and three children. All are given the same love, affection, and education and yet each one will turn out to be an individual personality. One may turn out to be a doctor, another an artist, and the third may still be trying to find himself long after the others have graduated from college and entered upon careers. We can only say at this point that we have not found the perfect formula for predicting human behavior, and why should we want such a stage of development? Living with a certain amount of uncertainty is healthy for us. To digress a moment, if you were asked the question, "Do you want to know the exact year, month, and day that you are going to die?" the majority of people would respond with a negative answer. We would rather take our chances and not have someone say, "An hour from now you will be dead."

To get back to our subject, the child as he grows quickly responds to everything around him. Life is constantly filled with frustrations and disappointments, big and small. The growing child must respond to these and take them in stride. The stronger the image he has built of his body the more easily he can handle these problems. To reiterate—a child growing up in a warm and trustful atmosphere has the odds going for him.

Growing up is not easy, even as the struggle to live is not easy. Life consists of ups and down. We must be able to take all of these changes in stride and still stay on top.

We must remember that at *each* stage of life we are now encrusted with everything that has happened before. The impact of all our experiences will be crucial to making decisions that affect the present. Since all of this is an ongoing thing, our body image is constantly shaping and re-shaping itself.

The news media shapes how we think about ourselves. A story comes out in the press about Governor John D. Rockefeller IV of West Virginia. Of course they report that he is rich but they also report that he is a "towering" six foot six and a half inches tall. He *must* be an overpowering figure. If we constantly keep hearing and reading these remarks, we will consider them to be true.

As a youngster reaches the adolescent stage, change and growth become rapid. Not only physical growth but mental growth, too—think of all the decisions a 14 through 17 year old must make. He must cope with a rapidly changing body and relate to his peers in a positive way. He has a desire for independence and yet is dependent. He also must think ahead. Before long he will be graduating from high school, but in grades 9, 10, and 11—three short years—he must make decisions that may affect him for the rest of his life. What subjects should he take in high school? Should he plan on college? Will he have the money to attend? How about the girl friend or boy friend?

So many problems, so many decisions and yet so few years to cope with them.

Now we are talking about what we conceive as a perfectly normal youngster, but how about the one who has a physical handicap. And we are not talking about big handicaps. How about the youngster who wears glasses and has buck teeth but otherwise is in perfect physical condition? These two problems can have a tremendous impact, perhaps giving the youngster an inferiority complex that may be very difficult to overcome. Yet there are solutions to the problem. For a girl or boy, contact lenses may be the answer to the problem of glasses. A visit to the dentist may be the answer to the problem of faulty teeth. It is amazing how these problems, once corrected, will completely change an individual. Frequently people, no matter what their age, are not aware that certain physical characteristics or habits may be hampering them. Your best friend is not the one who fails to tell you about your problem. Others can frequently see you better than you can see yourself. The one who can tell you, in a tactful way, that you have bad breath is doing you more of a service than the one who lets you keep going with this condition.

We live in an inside world and an outside world. Let us examine this. What is happening inside of you, the hormone changes, sex changes, and growth changes, happen in such a way that we are not even aware of them, but the outside world is having its impact also. It is bombarding our body and our body is reacting to this stimuli.

One problem that adolescents have, for example, is acne. Why is this happening? Here is the inside world now working more rapidly. The glands that regulate the growth have speeded up. Oil secretion has increased and this in turn may cause blackheads and pimples.

Now a boy or girl with pimples must face the external world. Adolescents are quick to pick up the signals of possible disapproval from their peers. The girl does not get dates. Everything else about her is great, but oh! that pimply face. The image she now has of herself changes. Depending on the severity of the problem we may get a mild withdrawal to a very severe withdrawal from life. Some will try to compensate by studying harder and using their time in this constructive way.

Everything concerning how a person handles a problem has to be involved within the context of the environment or setting in which a person lives. If you are in a certain social circle, tattoos on the body are perfectly acceptable. And for many young men, the tattoo is a signal of masculinity and a heightened self-image.

In the context of the self-image of one's body, not every part of the body is given equal status. In our society, one's stature or height is considered very significant. The short person is really on the short end of the stick in terms of social approval. This is especially true of men. One's legs are also significant but for different reasons for boys and girls. For a girl, her legs are part of an attractive sexual armour. She may not have much of a face but if she has beautiful legs, this feature may well compensate for other characteristics which may be less attractive.

But styles and what we consider attractive may change. Consider the popularity of long hair for boys. In a very short period of time, it became the style for almost all males. One modeled his hair, beard, and clothes after a stereotype model. One's self-image improved if he could come close to this ideal model.

There is nothing wrong in building our body image on what we consider ideal types. When we model ourselves on perfect body types, which would include the finest in physical, mental, and spiritual qualities, we are in effect enhancing our own. The power that exists in that individual will now become incorporated into our own. We have, so to speak, internalized an ideal figure as part of our own. The power that exists in that individual will now become a powerful influence on our own life. The determination and body force needed to overcome obstacles in life will be enhanced. Selecting an ideal type for ourselves is a positive approach to life.

But if one looks back we can find many individuals who have distorted bodies and yet made contributions to our society of an outstanding nature. Such a person, for example, was Charles Steinmetz, the electrical wizard. He was almost barred from entering the country because of his dwarflike, hunchback body. But eventually he was employed by the General Electric Company and made contributions in the field of electricity that were sheer works of genius.

So, individuals can overcome obstacles and make contributions that enhance the life style of all of us.

It is unfortunate, though, that so many believe what others say about them or what they perceive is being said about them, that they incorporate someone else's image of them, which may be incorrect. These people are simply accepting values which they think are correct and then in ways subtle and not so subtle impose them on the rest of us. Again, height is extremely important, especially for men.

No one stays an infant or an adolescent, forever. Life moves inexorably onward. Before long we have reached middle age. The hormonal system and the basal metabolism system are still working, but you are not at 45 what you were at 25. For the woman, the hormonal system is changing. She is now entering the phase of menopause. Her physical characteristics are changing. The estrogen level is dropping. As the woman gets older, a process of osteoporosis begins to work. This means that the bones become more porous. There is also a softening of the bone. Up to 2 inches in height may be lost. A hump at the upper spine will be noticeable—popularly called the "dowager's hump." All of these changes that occur have a tremendous effect upon a person's view of his body image. We can accept the changes that are taking place and even slow down the process by changing our diet, improving our nutritional intake, and taking advantage of all the latest research that has been done with relation to vitamins and minerals. We must take a realistic, not pessimistic, view of life.

The situation that applies to women, also applies to men. Decreasing ability to see, the wearing of bifocal lenses, less body agility, sagging jowls, and wrinkled skin can all have a damaging effect on our body image.

And it may be that your personal view of yourself may be more damaging than any glandular changes that are taking place. You can dress in a style appropriate to your age and make use of all the modern devices and cosmetics that will enhance your body image. You don't have to walk around without teeth. Make use of anything that improves that personal picture of yourself that is positive and strong.

Losing the function of any part of our body can have a dramatic influence on our entire outlook on life. Take the case of Jerry Wall. *The Arizona Daily Star* reported that he was despondent because he would have to have his right leg amputated. He had had a diabetic ulcer which had at first cost him his toes and, then, the eventual amputation of the entire leg. After the amputation he was even more depressed. All sorts of feelings welled up in him about what a one-legged man could do and how he would react. And then he read a story about Jim O'Harra, who was a policeman in Tucson. Jim had lost a part of his leg. Jim O'Harra recovered and is now a full-time policeman.

Jerry contacted police headquarters in Tucson, Arizona and was surprised to get a personal visit from Jim O'Harra. Jim went directly to his room at the Tucson Medical Center and talked directly to Jerry. He answered all of his questions and showed him his artificial limb. In effect, Jim was a model for Jerry. Jerry's spirits brightened and he now displays a new spirit of independence.

Heart attack! The very thought will send a cringe of fear down our spine and may result in a permanent change of body image in some. The heart has a way of being viewed as the central part of not only our body but of our emotional life. There is only one heart. If that stops, life stops. And is it any wonder that the individual perhaps in the prime of his life—the thirties or forties—may be suddenly struck down. He may be working as a successful salesman, but his earnings depend upon his being out in the field and earning his commission. He now feels the pressure of not only being unable to work but of, perhaps, being permanently crippled. He wonders about his job. Will his employer consider him a "has been"? Anxiety and fear permeate his personality. Problems of being unable to sleep may develop. How will his wife and children view him?

And yet, let us take a look at another side of this situation. One which I think will amaze the majority of readers. Let us tell you the story of a program that is in progress in Honolulu.

First, answer this question: If you, the average person, could run the 26-mile marathon, would you consider yourself to be in pretty good shape? Would you believe that they have a cardiac rehabilitation program in Honolulu for heart attack victims and the graduation exercise is to run the 26-mile marathon? Imagine what *that* does to your body image, not to mention the improvement in your body health that this program has resulted in.

Jo Schroeder, R.N., M.S., reported on how the program works in *R.N.*, a professional journal. The program in Honolulu is so interesting that it bears study. A healthy, strong and fit body has to be an asset to our body image and exercise is such an important aspect that our readers may want to know about the Honolulu program.

Every December a marathon run is sponsored in Honolulu. Men and women of all ages including heart attack patients are in the crowd of runners. The cardiac patient is gradually eased into the running program. The patient's progress is constantly monitored. Gradually, the patient acquires a new life style and body image. It is not easy to make these changes. One must give up smoking, adopt correct nutritional habits, and exercise on a regular basis. The nurses who supervise the exercise program are also marathon runners. The patients who follow the program which takes many months to complete are 97% successful in completing the marathon. An interesting question: Why not just jogging? According to the author, joggers who run less than six miles still die from coronary heart disease. The author reports that there have been no documented deaths from coronary heart disease among the marathon runners—regardless of heart problems or age. The author reports on 54-year-old Tommy R. They called him the "3-Clogged-Arteries Kid" because three coronary arteries were plugged up—85, 95, and 99%. Tom had to make a decision—surgery or exercise.

He chose exercise. One year later Tommy has successfully completed three marathons.

Author Jo Schroeder says the "real miracle" occurs when the 26-mile run is completed. One can well image the positive feeling a person has about his body when such a strenuous endurance test is completed.

Our body image extends beyond our body, *per se*. The car one drives, the clothes we wear, the cosmetics we use, our jewelry, furniture, neighborhood, and how and where we work —all of this is part of our image.

When we see a person clothed in a certain fashion, our mind quickly forms a certain view. The nurse in her uniform projects an image as does the policeman.

Individuals have a heightened worth of themselves when they feel well-dressed. When you go to a formal dance, and you are attired in an attractive evening gown, you have that feeling of being on top of the world.

Designers of clothes have the sexual appeal of clothes in mind. That which has an erotic appeal enhances the item of clothing. Proper clothing and various symbols placed in strategic places will enhance sexual appeal on the part of the opposite sex and also create envy and admiration from those of the same sex.

The marriage ceremony from beginning to end is an extension of an idealized body image. The bride in gown, the entire bridal entourage, the fancy limousine, the grand dining room, and all the other beautiful trappings surrounding this ceremony tend to inflate one's feelings about himself or herself and also to stamp this event as a most memorable occasion.

The executive sitting behind an impressive desk is trying to project himself as an important person. He steps into the chauffered limousine to further his image. Up and down the line this sort of playacting goes on. Everyone, in one way or another, is involved in this game.

14. The Mind

At the center of our body image is our mind. The human mind is the most magnificent creation in the entire universe. Your mind is the generator of ideas which can eventually become reality. And the kind of reality you want can be determined by you. We are aware of all the forces that move us in one direction or another, and maybe we can't change everything, but we can start positive movement that will make us happier and feel in balance with the nature of things.

You don't have to live with negative feelings about yourself. To change is not easy but one can change.

All of the magnificent buildings and bridges, every invention, was once an idea or dream in someone's mind. But one just couldn't dream about it. Action on that dream had to be taken. And that takes effort, work, and sweat. The dream is the easy part—it is the follow-through that is most important.

Ralph Waldo Emerson captured the essence of human qualities in his essay on *Self-Reliance*—he urges us to believe our own thoughts:

> "To believe your own thought, to believe that what is true for you in your private heart, is true for all men—that is genius."

Emerson urges us to harness the power that is within us. You won't know that power until you try it out.

"Trust thyself," he says. How many of us lack the confidence of our thoughts. And Emerson also urges us not to be afraid of making mistakes. Suppose you contradict yourself—so what!

Consistency is the hobgoblin of little minds, he says. He urges us to speak what we think in hard words and tomorrow speak what tomorrow thinks in hard words again, though it may contradict everything you said today. So you are misunderstood—weren't Socrates, Jesus, Luther, Galileo, and Copernicus misunderstood? Those who bring a new idea that may shake up a cozy style of living are frequently looked upon with suspicion. Yet every day every one of us is constantly changing. New adjustments must be made to accommodate the changed situation.

We should constantly keep our mind focused on the idea that we are equal to the best of humanity that has ever existed.

Walt Whitman, one of America's greatest poets, sums it up thus:

> The messages of great poets to each man and woman are, Come to us on equal terms, Only then can you understand us, We are no better than you, What we enclose you enclose, What we enjoy you may enjoy. Did you suppose there could be only one Supreme? We affirm there can be unnumbered Supremes, and that one does not countervail another . . . and that men can be good or grand only of the consciousness of their supremacy within them. What do you think is the grandeur of storms and dismemberments and the deadliest battles and wrecks and the wildest fury of the elements and the power of the sea and the motion of nature and of the throes of human desires and dignity and hate and love? It is that something in the soul which says, Rage on, Whirl on, I tread master here and everywhere, Master of the spasms of the sky and of the shatter of the sea. Master of nature and passion and death, And of all terror and all pain.

15. Exercise and Activity Chart

SOME individuals find it convenient to keep a daily record of what they do—exercises that they engage in or various activities that involve them such as club dates, church attendance or classes they attend. In fact, one may want to keep systematic evidence of how much one eats, smokes, drinks, works, and even the mood one is in each day.

The chart that follows is just a general guide. You should really arrange it to your own particular needs; you can put dates in as suits your particular requirement. Some may find it convenient to keep a large chart on the wall at home.

You can put a large chart on your bedroom wall so that when you awaken you just won't fail to be reminded about what to do and you'll have no excuse for not writing everything down. Write on the chart exactly how you felt the moment you got up and make yourself a written promise for that day that you'll keep a record of everything significant bearing on your health and well-being for that day. Also keep a small note-book in your pocket to record data throughout the day and then post it on the chart at a convenient time. If you follow this procedure, you will have a consistent record of what is happening to you as an individual over a period of time.

You may be on a weight-reducing program. Before you hit the refrigerator for that snack, make it a point to first note the snack on the chart or in the notebook. Doing this may very well act as a deterrent to eating. You will have given yourself a second thought. Actually, you'll find this an effective method of cutting down on eating between meals. The chart is a desirable and objective way of carrying on a continuous program of self-examination.

Actually, the idea of keeping a catalog of one's daily activities is not new. Benjamin Franklin felt that a ledger of his life would be very helpful. When Ben Franklin made out his chart, he was thinking in terms of moral perfection, but in a way he was trying to conform to what he thought was an ideal or perfect form. When we try to improve ourselves it is because we initially sense that there is part of us that does not meet what we feel as ideal.

Use your chart as a total plan for the day or a longer period of time. If you have mapped a certain day for food shopping, post a little message to eat before you go. This will cut down on the impulse buying of many food items. An empty stomach is a poor guide to successful shopping.

Of course, you can also follow Ben Franklin's example and list the virtues that he liked to keep tabs on, such as temperance, order, and frugality. Ben Franklin arranged his virtues in a certain order and temperance was at the top of his list.

Exercise Number

	1	2	3	4	5	6	7	8	9	10
1st Day										
2nd										
3rd										
4th										
5th										
6th										
7th										
8th										
9th										
10th										
11th										
12th										

Figure 48